Principles and Practices of
Contamination Control and Cleanrooms

Principles and Practices of

Contamination Control and Cleanrooms

C. K. Moorthy

PharmaMed Press
An imprint of Pharma Book Syndicate
A unit of BSP Books Pvt. Ltd.
4-4-309/316, Giriraj Lane,
Sultan Bazar, Hyderabad - 500 095.

Third Reprint 2019

C K Moorthy
Founder & Principal Facilitator
Center for GMP
49 Aruna Enclave Trimulgherry, Secunderabad 500015
Voice: 27791629 **Fax:** 27992912
eMail: cgmp@vsnl.com **URL:** business.vsnl.com/cgmp

Published by

PharmaMed Press
An imprint of Pharma Book Syndicate
A unit of BSP Books Pvt. Ltd.
4-4-309/316, Giriraj Lane, Sultan Bazar, Hyderabad - 500 095.
Phone: 040-23445600, 23445688; Fax: 91+40-23445611
E-mail: info@pharmamedpress.com
www.pharmamedpress.com/pharmamedpress.net

ISBN: 978-93-86819-60-4 (Hardbound)

Dedicated to

Sri C M Shahani,
whose passion for the subject inspired my own;
and to those researchers and workers, renowned and unknown, whose contributions, large and small, have helped nudge the frontiers of Microcontamination Control & Biosafety even further

Success in contamination control
comes not from the absence of contaminants at the work space
but from the ability to cope with them

Contents

Preface

Microcontamination control has yet to evolve as a separate discipline. As a consequence, specialists in other fields are assigned responsibilities in this field. Information gaps naturally abound in the industry.

To illustrate, consider the questions on the following page. The answers are at the end of the book, and in between are the *whys*, *whats* and *hows*.

There is a dire need for a coherent reference book that offers insights, guidance and assistance to ensure that facilities, practices and procedures are in compliance with current norms. Sadly available information lies scattered and dispersed; and few publications exist that piece these nuggets together. Over the past decade participants at my training programs have been urging me to publish, so that the information I share finds a wider audience.

This book is my response. It is neither a treatise nor a survey of the subject neither a handbook nor a manual, it is merely an assemblage of my lecture notes aimed at closing some, if not all, of such gaps. As a happy result, the reader need not feel constrained to read from cover to cover or in any particular sequence. Each topic is dealt with under a separate section, and is by and large independent of the sections, preceding or succeeding.

Nevertheless the sequencing of the topics has been arranged with a view to develop the concept of an integrated microcontamination control and refine it as we go along. In that sense, the book would best serve its intended purpose if it were read in the same logical sequence.

As production volumes sky rocket, we shall be witnessing the disappearance of marginal players, and the emergence of strong, vibrant units with economy of scale. The challenge will lie in our ability to maintain consistency and uniformity in our product quality and value across multi-locational facilities to safeguard our reputation and profits. Failure will not be an option.

The material presented here has been obtained from people and published sources, too numerous to mention. My contribution is in stringing together such bits of data and representing them in a coherent, cogent, ready-to-use format.

This book restricts itself to applications where contaminant *exclusion* is the primary objective; not *containment*. Hence, hazardous operations requiring operator safety and environment protection are not touched upon. These are special cases calling for a radically different design approach, and the reader is referred to the authoritative guidelines available from sources such as CDC, NIH, OSHA, and LCDC.

- C. K. Moorthy

***What would you say: True* or *False* ?**

1. Cleanrooms are contaminant free environments.
2. A cleanroom is incomplete without an air shower.
3. HEPA filter is a 0.3 micron bacteria tight sieve. Larger particles are arrested; smaller particles escape.
4. Particle count at 0.5 micron or larger per cubic foot of air sampled immediately downstream of a properly installed new HEPA filter should always be 100 or better.
5. LAF refers to air moving at 90 fpm in parallel lines.
6. A HEPA can have an "acceptable" leak.
7. A HEPA may be repaired at site if the media is damaged.
8. It is not important whether the measurement is taken with a counter sampling at 0.01, 0.1 or 1 CFM, because readings are automatically extrapolated.
9. If airflow is reduced, pinhole leaks are detected more easily.
10. At the end of a properly validated sterilisation cycle all microorganism are killed.

1 Basics of Contamination Control

Contaminants play an especially important role in the manufacture, manipulation or repair of such items as semiconductors, space vehicles, conventional and nuclear missiles, microbial cultures, ball-bearings, parenterals, vaccines and human organs.

While it may be unusual to think of the human body as a product, or the Operation Theatre as a factory, the same engineering principles of microcontamination control apply. The control of infectious airborne pathogenic organisms in hospital operating rooms and recovery wards can be achieved in a manner identical to that used to protect against airborne contaminants during pattern generation

Users of Controlled Microenvironments Worldwide

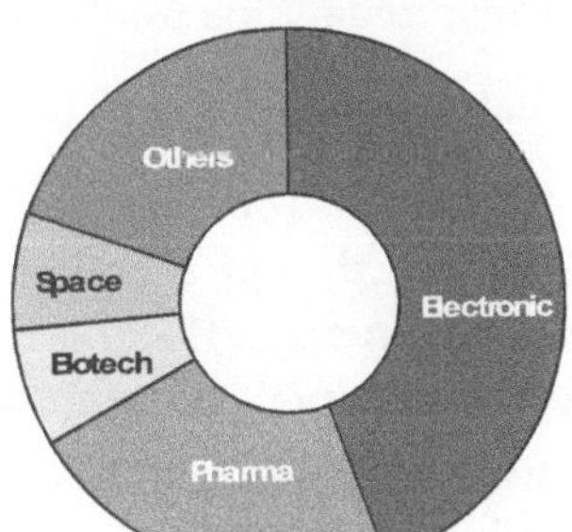

Fig. 1.1

of semiconductor devices, or during aseptic manipulations with thermolabile injectibles. The “risks” of manufacture, of course, are different since the loss of a human life has consequences beyond economics. But the technical approaches to solving the problem remain similar.

Contamination control is only a part of the larger Quality Assurance Initiatives that aim to minimise the risk of producing a defective, and maximise the probability of manufacturing a product "fit for use" or "fit for purpose". By this token, contamination control is best described as a set of systems, practices and procedures that aspire to minimise the introduction of a contaminant into a product or process.

Contamination control can be compared to providing the highest level of personal security to a VIP under threat. Depending on whether the VIP is the President of the United States of America, or of Sri Lanka, or of India, the group posing the threat differs. Once we know the identity of the VIP, we are better placed not only to anticipate the sources of the threat, but also to know more about their origin, locations, motives and modus operandi.

The security steps we normally take are:

1. Isolate the VIP
2. Minimise his exposure, both in terms of duration and frequency
3. Seek and destroy or immobilise those threatening his safety
4. If his enemies are outside, we make it difficult for them to penetrate the protective barriers
5. If they are already within, we flush them out
6. We monitor those in his immediate proximity
7. We advise the VIP not to antagonise anyone who may be around him, friend today, foe tomorrow (Don't *generate* enemies within)
8. Stay vigilant and cope

In the context of contamination control, a product or process is what we try to safeguard, and a contaminant is any substance or energy which produces an *adverse* effect on that product or process. Such a classification is purely contextual, without bearing on its absolute worth. Just as the enemy of one VIP may not necessarily be an enemy of the next VIP, so too in contamination control. Light is precious for all of us, but not for photoprocessing; gold, too, is precious, but not a speck is welcome in the wrong place on a wafer.

Contamination control measures make more sense once we understand contaminants and the contamination process.

Contaminant Classification

Regarded from the stand point of the 'type' of *damage* they do, contaminants may be divided into subgroups :

Table1.1

SUBSTANCE			ENERGY
Physical	Chemical	Biologic	
Dust Dirt Grit Fibre Lint Fly ash	Organic compounds Inorganic salts Vapour Mist Fume Smoke	Bacteria Fungus Spore Pollen Virus Human skin cells	Thermal Light Electromagnetic (EMI) Electrostatic (ESD) Radiation Electrical (RF)

- ***Physical :*** Particles that cause damage by virtue of their *physical properties* alone: for example, a grain of sand can score a bearing, or obstruct light in photoprocessing.
- ***Chemical :*** Organic chemicals such as oils, fats, waxes, fluxes, paints and plastics may *react chemically* with a product and change its properties, or simply insulate the product and interfere with its processing. Inorganic chemicals, being ionic by nature, modify the electrical characteristics of precision electronic products. Gases induce contamination (like oxidation) only in the gaseous phase. In contrast, vapours and mists contaminate in the vapour phase; on condensation, in the liquid phase (like oil films); and, on subsequent evaporation, in the solid phase (residues).
- ***Biological :*** Microorganisms are the critical contaminants in pharmaceuticals, biotechnology, food & beverage processing, cosmetics and patient care.
- ***Energy :*** Some products are thermolabile; some sensitive to electrostatic discharge (ESD); some are affected by RF & EMI.

Contaminant Pathway

If you were to ask any agency that provides security to VIPs they will tell you that the enemy may attempt a million times and fail; he needs to succeed just once. In contrast, they must succeed each time. This is just as true with contamination control.

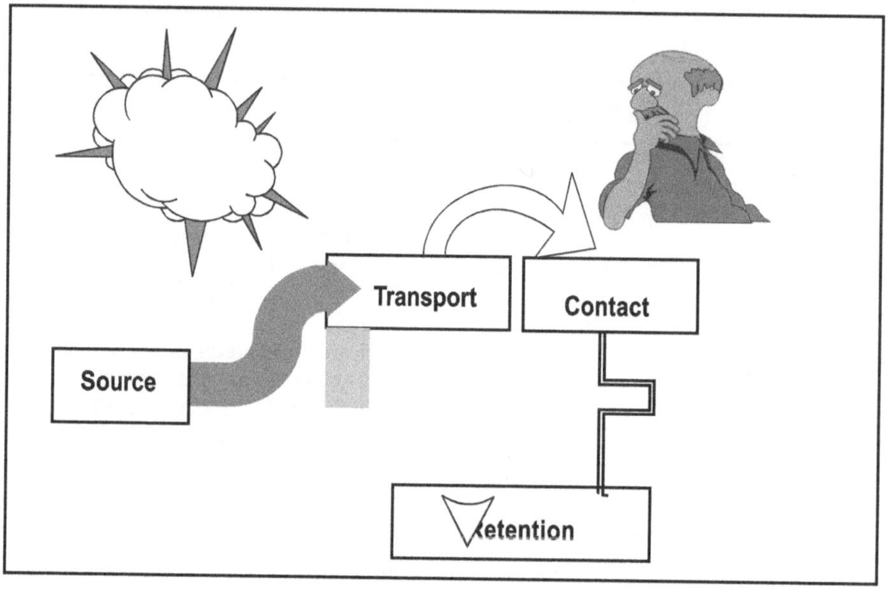

Fig. 1.2 The Contaminant Pathway

On the flip side, the mere presence of a contaminant does not automatically imply contamination. For contamination to occur, the contaminant must first have its *source*; must then be *transported* and reach the product site; must make *contact* with the product; and must be *retained* by the product.

If this process of contamination, known as the *contaminant pathway*, is broken at any stage, contamination does not occur.

For instance, if the source of the contaminant is absent; or, having a source, it is unable to access the product; or, having somehow managed to slip through, is prevented from making contact; or, even after having made contact, is not retained, or not allowed to be retained, *contamination does not take place*, and the product is safe.

Contamination control may then be viewed as an exercise that aims to break the contaminant pathway at one or more stages of the contamination process.

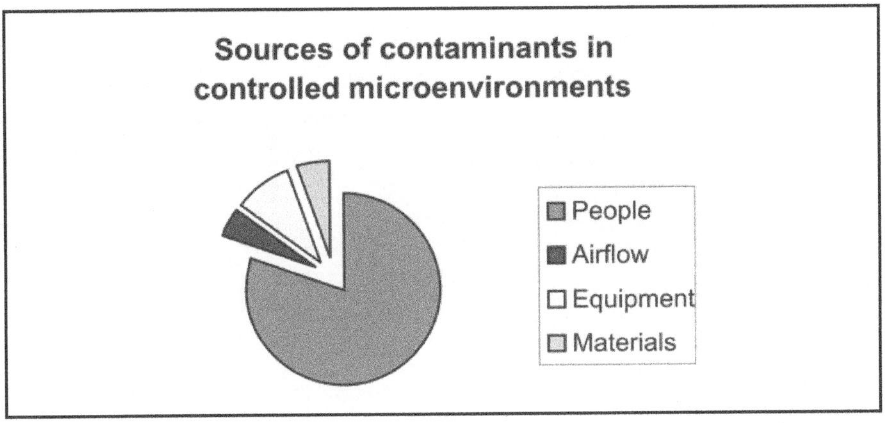

Fig. 1.3

Sources of Contaminants

Included contaminants emanate from raw materials and consumables; *fluidised* contaminants from utilities; *suspended* contaminants from the environment; *settled* contaminants from dust collecting surfaces; *emitted* contaminants from machinery, moving parts and surfaces; *shedded* and *transferred* contaminants from personnel.

In fact, research into a large number of reported occurrences of contamination in well-designed and maintained clean rooms reveals that in 5% of the cases it was due to *contaminated raw materials*; in 10% through *utilities* and *defective or soiled equipment, tools or implements*; in 5% due to *faulty air filtration;* and in 80% due to *breaches in the product-person interface.*

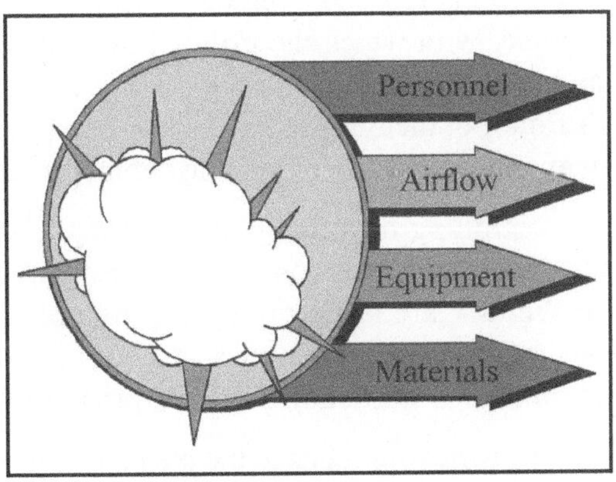

Fig. 1.4

Hence, contrary to popular belief, microcontamination control does not begin and end with air filtration: it is only one of many concurrent initiatives. Comprehensive microcontamination control requires a program that effectively integrates and orchestrates planned offensive

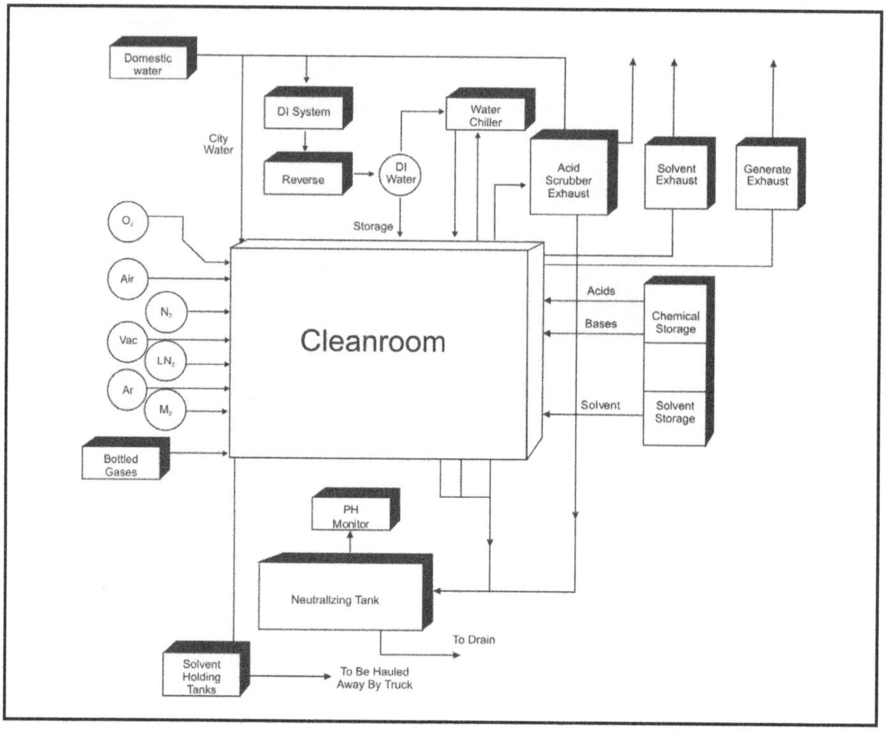

Fig. 1.5 Typical Semiconductor Processing Facility

measures on all four fronts. Pursuing one while ignoring others yields sub-optimal results.

I have personally seen many facilities where such "common sense" is conspicuous by its absence. The User forces me through a commendable decontamination entry regimen, only to leave me watch in amazement the impunity with which the trolley boy "gate crashes" from the material entry; double-doored and air locked. No decontamination protocols apply to him, his trolley or their dirt-laden wheels, except on some neatly typed SOP, stashed away in the recesses of a filing cabinet in the Production Manager's Office.

Controlling the quality of incoming raw materials, consumables, liquids and gases, and selection and use of equipment and accessories appropriate for the task are subjects beyond the scope of this book. They have been mentioned to record that these avenues too must be looked into as sources of contaminants while drawing up a program for microcontamination control.

We restrict our focus to the management of contaminants that are airborne, and those at the product-person interface.

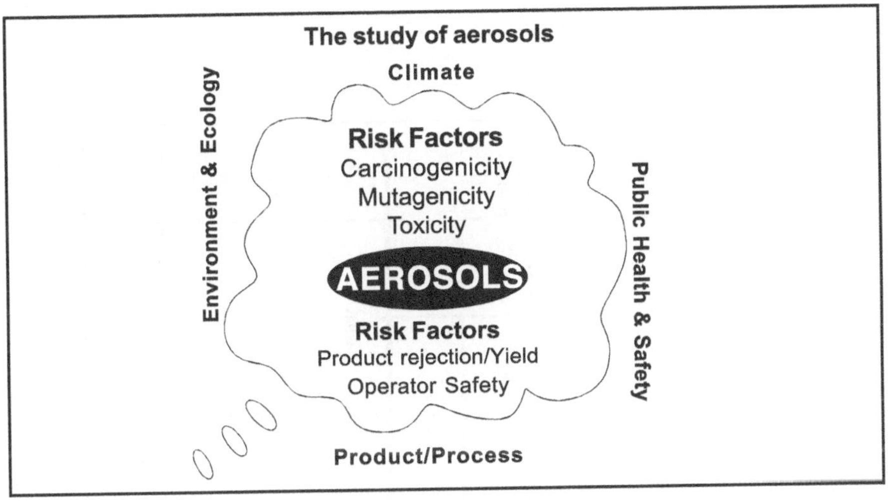

Fig. 1.6

Aerosols

The subject of aerosols has long interested researchers in pollution control as well as contamination control. In the former group are those in Public Health who worry about the risk factors associated with atmospheric pollution; environment scientists who are concerned about adverse ecological effects; and meteorologists whose interest is in determining the influence on climate

Table 1.2

Number of Particles/m³ in Outdoor Air			
Size µm	Dirty	Normal	Clean
>0.1	1×10^{10}	3×10^{9}	5×10^{8}
>0.3	3×10^{8}	9×10^{7}	2×10^{7}
>0.5	3×10^{7}	7×10^{6}	1×10^{6}

and weather, as a consequence of which a wealth of data is available. Our interest is in examining their potential to compromise product yield and operator safety.

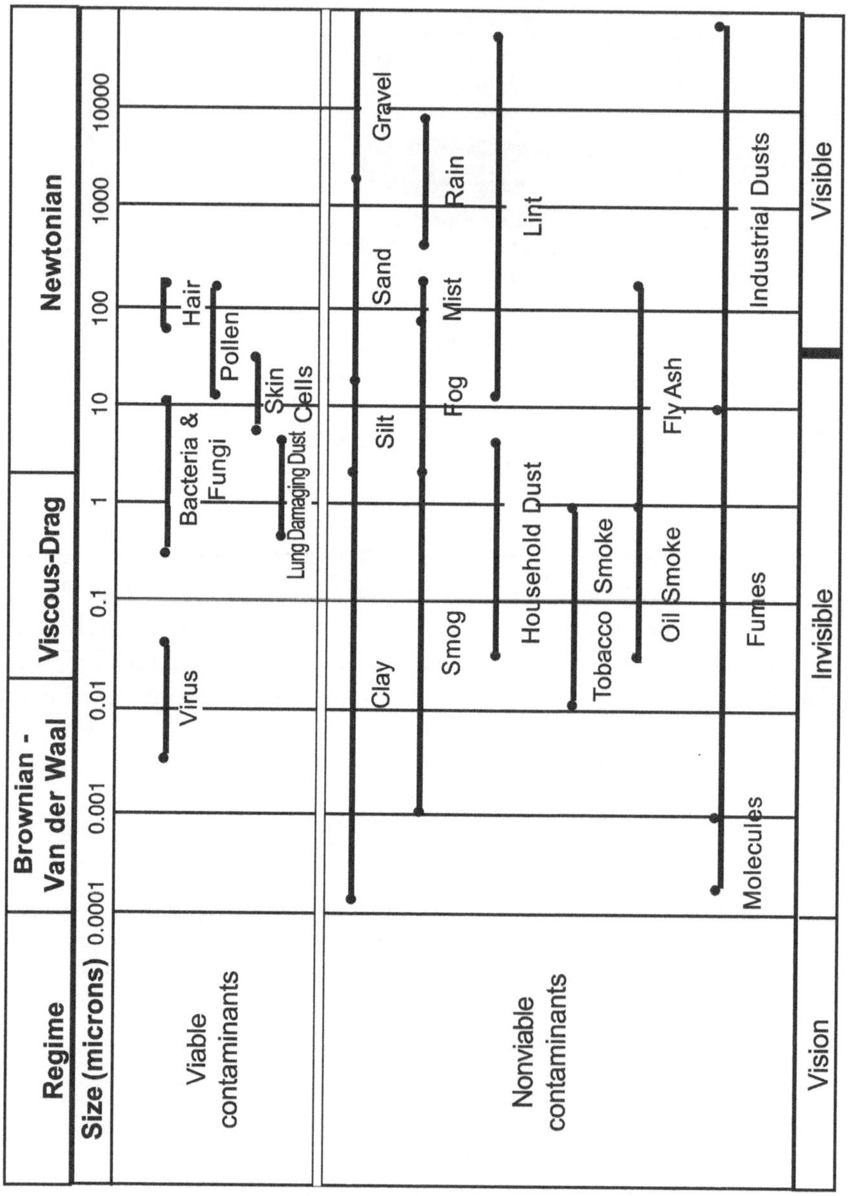

Fig 1.7 Size Distribution of typical suspended contaminants

The conventional unit of measurement for suspended particles is the micron (μ), or one-millionth part of a metre. To have some idea of the relative sizes, it may be noted that the diameter of average human hair is 100μ. Rain is a good example of 1000μ suspended droplets that settle out quickly, attaining a terminal velocity much before they reach ground level. Human vision with the unaided eye stops at 50μ.

Suspended Particulate Regimes

Larger particles have a relatively short "life" as *suspended* contaminants, and settle out rapidly. This is due to the fact that those in size above 20μ have sufficient mass to respond to gravity. Such particles are referred to, for the purpose of this discussion, as *Newtonian* particles or particles belonging to the *gravitational regime*. (Since our vision is limited to 50μ, this means that visible particles do not remain suspended in aerosols; in other words, the particles that do remain suspended in the aerosol are too small to be seen. Suspended contaminants are, therefore, by and large invisible. In fact, in an average cleanroom, 97% of suspended contaminants are sub-visible).

Particles in the size range 0.1μ to 10μ do not have sufficient mass for gravitational forces to be effective; they respond, instead, to *viscous drag forces* and move with air currents. We refer to these as *Stokes-Cunningham* particles or particles belonging to the *drag regime*.

Particles smaller than 0.1μ, and approaching molecular sizes, hardly have any mass, and are too small even for viscous pulls and pushes. They are in a constant state of Brownian motion, the irregular movement of suspended particles as a result of bombardment by atoms and molecules, Van der Waal forces, electrostatic attraction and repulsion. We call these *Brownian* particles or particles in the *diffusion regime*. As mentioned earlier, every single suspended contaminant in the aerosol is not necessarily a threat to the product. In order to contaminate, it must *first reach* the product. Let us therefore study the different mechanisms at play that can propel a contaminant toward the critical work area and precipitate the deposition process.

Gravitational Propulsion

If the particle is *newtonian*, gravity is probably the most recognised mechanism for particle movement and deposition. Particles in any liquid or gas of a lower density will settle out, reaching a terminal velocity determined by the balance between gravitational forces and the viscous drag of the fluid. Contaminants above the work site have the potential to reach the product while settling down. On the other hand, if the particle is below product datum level, it cannot cause harm as long as it remains at that level.

Table 1.3 Velocity of settling of typical suspended contaminants

Diameter of particles (microns)	Velocity of settling: Feet per minute	Velocity of settling: Inches per hour	Velocity of settling: Centimetres per second	Regime	Transport
< 0.02	?	?	?	Brownian-Van der Waal	Diffusion
0.05	0.00003	0.022	0.000015	Viscous-Drag	Air currents
0.1	0.00016	0.115	0.000081		
0.2	0.00036	0.259	0.00018		
0.4	0.0013	0.936	0.00066		
0.8	0.005	3.6	0.0025		
1	0.007	5.04	0.0036		
2	0.024	17.4	0.012		
5	0.2	144	0.102		
10	0.59	425	0.3		
20	2.4	1,728	1.2		
40	9.5	6,840	4.8		
60	21.3	15,320	10.8	Newtonian	Gravity
80	37.9	27,250	19.2		
100	352	253,500	179		
400	498	360,000	253		

Similarly, a particle of sufficient mass moving in a fluid may find it difficult to negotiate deviating flow lines, specially when the fluid flows around obstacles in the course. In the process of bypassing the obstacle its momentum may cause it to veer out of control and cut across the flow to impinge and settle on the boundary wall. Or it may collide, lose momentum, and fall out. These are *inertial* mechanisms.

Sedimentation is a process triggered by the balance between gravity and forces of uniform fluid flow causing a suspended contaminant to settle out in a parabolic trajectory. The linear distance travelled is a function of fluid velocity and particle weight. The mass dependence of inertial forces reduces their influence in the sub-newtonian size range.

Drag Propulsion

Air currents are the principal cause of spread of suspended *Stokes-Cunningham* particles through their vigorous mixing action: the greater the air velocity and turbulence, the wider the range of spread. This phenomenon could facilitate drag regime particles to reach the product from any location or level in the room. (Liquids are more dense and viscous than air; hence fluidised particles are dragged over longer distances. If the contaminant dissolves, the dispersion and spread is even more pronounced).

Theoretical and experimental study of *turbulent* air currents is difficult, and little is known about the motion of particles suspended in turbulent flow. Particles will drop out no doubt; but the eddy currents present make it difficult to predict when, where or in which direction. All that can be said with any certainty is that the deposition rate will be an exponential decay function and that the velocity of any suspended particulate could be in any direction and of any magnitude.

Closely related to the concepts of turbulent flow are the *convection* currents in the environment. If there is a convective movement of gas containing suspended particles, there will be an interaction of forces between the gas medium and the particles tending to transport the particles on a bulk basis. Atmospheric clouds are examples of the convection phenomenon where droplets of water are transported great distances as a unit because of the temperature and concentration gradients between the cloud and the surrounding atmosphere.

Table 1.4

Regime	Brownian	Viscous-Drag	Newtonian
Propulsion medium	Assorted small particle effects	Air currents	Gravity
Regime-dependent deposition mechanism	Diffusion Electrostatic effects Capillary action Adsorption Van der Waal forces Coalescence Agglomeration	Surface tension	Sifting Sedimentation Inertial Forces
Regime-independent deposition mechanism	Impaction Interception Fibrillation Contaction	Impaction Interception Fibrillation Contaction	Impaction Interception Fibrillation Contaction

Artificial *agitation*, caused by personnel movements and process machinery motions, can, with the aid of the currents induced by the air distribution system in the room, transport suspended contaminants over considerable distances and precipitate deposition. The complex interplay of the mechanisms described above render it difficult to establish guidelines for the effects of 'artificially' induced agitation.

Diffusion Propulsion

Brownian motion causes spread of suspended ultrafines through diffusion: the higher the temperature, concentration, or diffusion coefficient, the larger the area of spread. The product could be compromised by a brownian particle from just about anywhere in the room.

Particles with diameter smaller than 0.1μ often grow in size till they assume a critical mass sufficient to settle out or be dragged away. Small particles tend to come together due to various mechanisms. Oppositely charged particles meet and become, neutral, but larger particles. While bombarding each other, two particles do not always rebound; if the Van der Waal force of intermolecular attraction is sufficiently strong, they stay bound together. In some cases a particle impinging on another loses its kinetic energy on impaction and remains loosely adhered at the surface. The first two are instances of *coalescence* where particles fuse together to form a larger particle; the last is an example of *agglomeration*. Both phenomena lead to cluster formations, and the cluster behaves exactly as a single homogeneous particle of that size would: either respond to gravity or to viscous drag forces.

Electrostatic charge can influence particle transport and deposition depending on the type of charge carried by the particle and the intensity of the electric or magnetic field present.

Other Mechanisms

Some deposition mechanisms are independent of particle size or the regime generally governing their behaviour. One of them is *impaction*, where a particle collides with and deposits on the surface of an obstructing object. Or, a particle could be *entrapped*, *occluded* or *enmeshed*, when its physical size precludes its passage through a porous obstacle. Similarly, if a suspended particle in motion encounters a series of obstacles that "trip" it in succession, it may lose sufficient kinetic energy and settle out, a mechanism known as *interception*.

Perhaps the most commonly occurring deposition is through *contaction*. Settled contaminants reach the product through the operator or any article or implement that makes physical contact with it while working.

With so many diverse forces and mechanisms at play, the 97% of sub-visible suspended contaminants in aerosols, left to themselves, tend to move about randomly, in all directions. But once we fully understand these influences, we are better equipped to devise methods to control and direct their trajectories out of harm's way.

The techniques developed in this book are directed more towards control of suspended particulates and microflora. However, moisture and airborne molecular contaminants (AMC) are also airborne, but require very special techniques for their management. Humidity is relatively better known, understood and controlled, but here we pause to get acquainted with airborne molecular contaminants.

Molecular contaminants

Although AMC is most commonly associated with the microelectronics, it is a problem in other processes such as spray painting, which have embraced cleanroom practices. In microelectronics, the shrinking chip geometry with

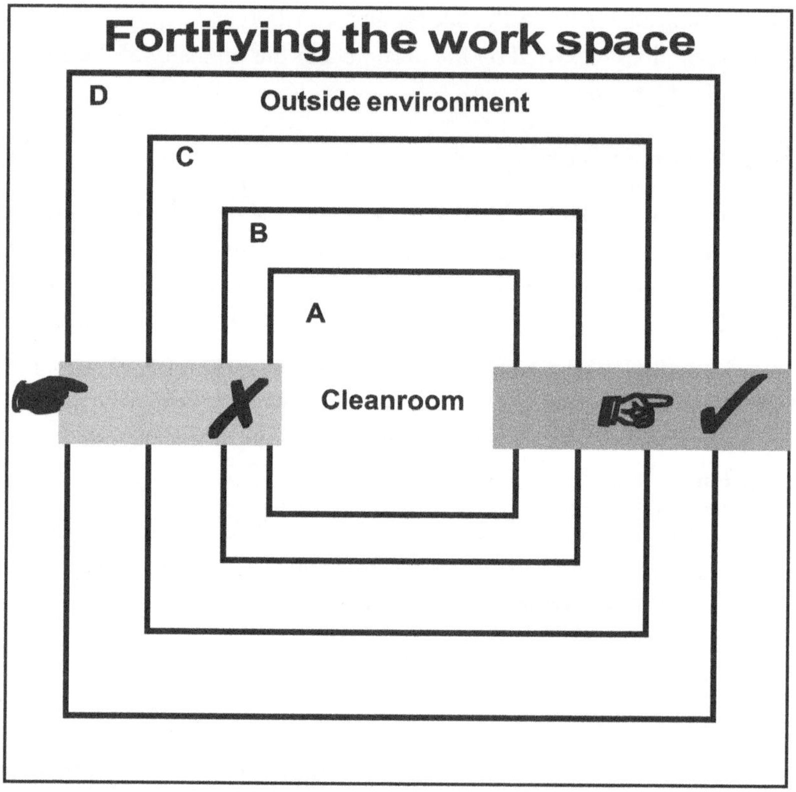

1 Identify the contaminant
2 Anticipate the contaminant
3 Prevent ingress
4 Facilitate egress
5 Minimise internal generation
6 Control residual contaminants

Fig. 1.8: The master plan for contamination control

critical sizes approaching molecular sizes is driving the need for testing and minimising AMC.

The AMC in cleanrooms may be classified as A, B, C and D (Acids, Bases, Condensables, and Dopants). The levels at which they are present in cleanrooms are often at the detection limits of instruments. In microelectronics, limits for molecular contamination as low as 0.1 ppt are forecast.

Current practice for controlling AMC is cleanrooms has taken a dual track. One is traditional practice of removal with gaseous filters or scrubbers. The other approach is to minimize or eliminate the use of materials that out gas the undesirable AMC. This has required clean materials for filter manufacture such as PTFE membranes, non boron or phosphor containing products, inert sealing compounds, and separators.

Of the AMC, in microelectronics, boron and organophosphates and their compounds are of main concern. Both boron and organophosphates are semiconductor dopants, and can diffuse into the silicon causing changes to the dopant level and electrical properties of the semiconductor. In other applications such as spray painting, silicone is a major concern.

Microfiber glass is suspected to be the primary source of boron in cleanrooms. In many cases, concentrations of ambient boron are high enough to make it nearly impossible to measure levels of boron from cleanroom filter media. Currently, boron in glass media is measured by extraction in water and reported as bulk concentration.

In cleanroom filters, the sources of organic compounds are the potting compounds used to seal the filter media to the filter frame, materials used for pleat separation, gaskets, and materials used in the manufacture of the media. Organophosphates are common fire retardants and are used widely in many potting and sealing compounds.

Of the organics, only the semi volatile compounds (with boiling points approximately between 100 to 400 ^{0}C) are of concern in materials of construction of cleanroom filters. The low boiling point materials are volatile enough to be eliminated rapidly at room temperatures. The higher boiling point materials are for the most part not gaseous at operating temperatures and are not a problem.

The current consensus for measuring the off gassing of the medium boiling point materials is to collect the materials in ambient air sampling tubes. The sampling tubes contain appropriate adsorbents to trap the compounds of interest. The sampling tubes are then analyzed by thermal desorption GC/MS. This method is also known as dynamic head space analyses. The sample is typically desorbed continuously at an elevated temperature while being purged by nitrogen. The out gassed compounds are then captured in a trap and analyzed by a GC/MS. The test provides only a relative abundance of the material in comparison to a reference. The temperature of the test can greatly affect the off gassing. It is a compromise between the higher temperatures needed to drive out more of the condensable from the material, and the lower temperatures needed to prevent the destruction of materials of interest. Currently, there is no consensus on the appropriate test temperature.

The master plan for contamination control

As mentioned at the outset, contamination control is much alike protecting a VIP, and the steps outlined for security apply here.

A product or process is susceptible to contamination during manufacture, assembly, testing, cleaning, transportation, storage or even while being used. Our objective is to minimise the risk of its being contaminated along the way.

Identifying the Contaminant

Our first exercise is in identifying the possible contaminants that threaten the product or proccss. Wc can then design a contamination control program that takes into account their characteristics and behavioural pattern.

Anticipting the Contaminant

Having identified the contaminants that are likely to compromise our product or process, we focus on the possible sources from where they could originate; and their mode of getting to the critical zone.

Preventing Ingress

Preventing ingress of contaminants into the selected work area. Since this book does not attempt to cover contaminants emanating from raw materials and utilities (*included* and *fluidised* contaminants), let us start with *suspended* contaminants. This is achieved by a combination of methods: controlling the particulate content through filtration of incoming air; isolating the product to the extent feasible from the harmful environment surrounding it; and entry restrictions with thorough decontamination of all materials, consumables, equipment, implements and personnel entering the zone. Where over pressurising is an available option, the balloon effect wards off incursions of suspended contaminants.

Table 1.5 : Basic microcontamination control checklist	
	Rigid inward Quality Control to check ingress of included contaminants through process raw materials/consumables, and fluidised contaminants through gases/liquids
Preventing Ingress	√ Select class of air cleanliness appropriate for the task √ Select location and layout optimising flowpaths for men, material and process ■ avoid loops in flowpaths ■ isolate through barriers ■ avoid direct / straight through access ■ stagger doorways ■ no windows on external wall ■ double-glazed view panels with breathers √ Sustain overpressure along clean-to-dirty axis, where not contraindicated √ Impose entry restrictions and thorough decontamination procedures for men, material and equipment
Facilitating Egress	√ Sustain overpressure along clean-to-dirty axis, where not contraindicated √ Avoid surfaces that can accumulate dust; where unavoidable, ensure easy accessibility to clean and disinfect √ Implement comprehensive sanitation plan
Minimising Generation	√ Select material and equipment that don't shed excessive particles or degas, especially walls, floor and ceiling √ Establish sound maintenance for upkeep of facility √ Operator training and discipline √ Good gowning
Coping with residual contaminants	√ Dilution of aerosol concentration by dilution: increase in air change rate √ Controlled velocity airflow without eddy currents to drag away suspended contaminants from critical zone: LAF √ Reduce product exposure time and exposure frequency

Since maintaining a high class of air cleanliness in the environment is always expensive, some designers advocate *task-specific* air cleanliness: a clean work bench in a cleanroom, where the air cleanliness at the work station is at least an order of magnitude higher than the surrounding environment.

Facilitating Egress

Facilitate egress of suspended as well as settled contaminants from within. The air distribution system should be designed to displace contaminated air to the exterior as directly and rapidly as possible. The principle of dilution can be employed: clean air can be passed through the given space in sufficient quantities to flush out as much of the contaminants generated within the space, and thinning out the concentration of the rest. An important corollary to control by dilution is an air distribution design that minimises recirculating eddy currents. An imaginative, effective and implementable sanitation scheme, closely supervised and monitored is another method of getting settled contaminants out of harm's way. Surfaces that gather dust should be avoided, or minimised where unavoidable; and all such surfaces should be smooth and accessible for thorough cleaning.

Minimising Internal Generation

Minimise generation of contaminants within. We start by reducing the number of operations, equipment, and personnel to the bare minimum. What can be done outside, must be done outside; what can be outside, should be outside; and who can be out side, should be outside. What remains inside is subjected to careful control: the process, equipment, operations and operator. As we shall see in a subsequent section, operator conduct and compliance often holds the key to successful contamination control.

Coping with Residual Contaminants

The last of the techniques relates to *coping with the residual contaminants*. Since deposition of suspended contaminants is a time dependent phenomenon, reducing *exposure frequency* and *exposure time* of sensitive products is an important form of control. Controlled eddy-free displacement of suspended contaminants, directed away from the critical site is another powerful method used to protect the product.

2 Environment Specification

We are now ready to specify the parameters for our clean room. But when we say clean do we really mean *clean*? Prima facie, clean implies absence of *soil*. Curiously we seldom use the word in its literal sense. Intuitively we understand the term in its relative sense. For example, a city is clean with plenty of clean parks, clean buildings and clean roads. And your clean crockery on your clean dining table in your clean home. Do we imply all are equally clean? No. The degree of soil we subconsciously discount is contextual to each case. That is why we would never set our buttered toast on the clean road, or perform surgery in the clean park. So how clean is *clean*?

To translate this qualitative concept to a quantifiable parameter for environment control, scientists measure the suspended contaminant density, or number of suspended particles per unit volume. The lower the contaminant density, the cleaner the environment.

We begin by determining or estimating the suspended contaminant density in a given room or at the work point of interest. Typically this lies in the range of 10 million (10^7) to 100 billion (10^{11}) per litre of atmospheric air. Ideally we would like to get rid of all of them. But that will cost money, and the proposition may not be financially viable. Fortunately, this extreme level of cleanliness is not warranted. Hence, we try to assess the maximum aerial contaminant density that the process can be carried out at risk levels that are acceptable and cost-effective: an environment "clean" enough for the intended purpose.

Classification of "air cleanliness"

Way back in 1963, the first "standard" was released in USA: US Federal Standard 209, which soon gained widespread acceptance as the primary document of reference for the semiconductor industry. Other nations and industries released their own standards and guidelines, which were more or less identical, except for minor differences in nomenclature and values. By 1992, when US Fed Std 209E was released, there were more than 300 cleanroom classification standards worldwide!

The absence of fine tuning specifications to the task on hand has been painfully acute: for example, we refer to *Air containing not more than 3.5 particles per litre or 100 particles per cubic foot of air sampled of size 0.5µ and larger*. But why "0.5µ"? It may have made eminent sense to the semiconductor industry where the minimal dimension (or line width) determines the maximum contaminant size. When the US Federal Standard 209 was being drafted, line widths hovered around 5µ , and statistics had established that a contaminant which is one-tenth in size has the potential to “kill”. Hence, the anchor at 0.5µ. But in Pharmaceuticals and Biotechnology, the threat is from microorganisms. Though they range in size from 0.3µ to 10µ, they seldom float free: almost without exception, they ride on a carrier particle, which is usually at least an order of magnitude larger. For example, almost all microorganisms in a cleanroom originate from people: skin scales and breath aerosols. Bacteria-laden particles or droplets in occupied rooms have an average equivalent diameter of approximately 12µ, which we know behave very differently from particles of size 0.5µ. The sedimentation rate for a 12µ particle is 0.46 cm/sec, and an occasional bacterium can deposit into a container, where the potential for multiplication is high.

It has been established that the level of microbial contamination of aseptic products is directly proportional to the aerial microbial concentration in the room. Though no universal relationship has yet been established between airborne contaminants and viable airborne contaminants, or between airborne bacteria-laden particles and airborne inanimate particles, there may be some situation-specific relationship.

In surgical suites there are reports that the ratio of viable to nonviable aerial contaminants is 1:1000. In Parenterals, it has generally been accepted in practice that an aerial microbial concentration of less than 20 CFU/cum is unlikely to cause deposition at the point of fill. These are nothing more than contentions based on conjectures. No statistically valid correlation has as yet been established.

But the need to specify simultaneously the acceptable levels of particles in the size ranges 3μ, 5μ, 10μ and 15μ, in addition to 0.5μ was recognised and acknowledged, and these concerns have been addressed by the new ISO standard 14644-1, where Macro-Particle density can be specified, and EUGGMP-2002, where the Microbial Limits are prescribed.

ISO 14698, issued in three parts, recommends a system for bioaerosol monitoring and control, but owing to the lack of consensus about what microorganisms are acceptable for whom, and what their concentration limits ought to be for which application, the standard stops short by merely stating that the User should define the target levels and derive the acceptable tolerance limits from that set point.

However, even though the limit for, say, 5μ particles is given, it is not realistic in practice to always achieve it or verify that it has indeed been achieved; and the zero count on 0.1 cft or even 1 cft samples can be very misleading. A much larger number of samples is needed to ascertain their density accurately. The difficulties mentioned here is touched in greater detail in the section on Qualification.

U S Federal Standard 209E

An important feature of US Federal Standard 209 (E) was its departure from the direction pursued by its predecessors. They not only defined air cleanliness classes, but also set values for other cleanroom parameters like air velocity, uniformity, parallelism, filter leak, decay, recovery, particle count, particle fall out rate, induction leaks, pressurisation, air supply capacity, air dilution rate, lighting, temperature, humidity, noise and vibration. The document contained comprehensive design data and facility guidelines. In contrast, the current version's focus is exclusively on air cleanliness and methods for verification. All other specifications are relegated to the vendor and buyer to mutually agree upon on the grounds that the technology is changing so rapidly and only the User can ascertain the parametric limits for his specific application, so that he gets a facility that is neither over-designed nor under-designed, but "fit for the intended purpose". Supplementary data is published by the Institute of Environmental Sciences under the title of Recommended Practices, where again the emphasis is on parametric testing and verification procedures rather than spelling out range values.

Recognising the fact that line widths in ULSIs have shrunk to submicronic levels, US Federal Standard 209 (E) introduced a new concept of U-descriptors to specify acceptable limits of aerosolised ultrafines. This refinement has been taken a step farther by the current ISO standard, which, as mentioned earlier, provides scope for specification of Macro-Particles.

But what does 0.5 micron mean? Diameter, length, breadth, width, depth, height, longest dimension, or average of all these? Suspended contaminants are predominantly irregular shaped. The amplitude of the electrical signal they induce in a photometer is compared with that produced by regular shaped objects in the same photometer, and the correspondence is deemed to be their ***equivalent diameter***.

The ISO family of Cleanroom Standards

Since the mother of all cleanroom technology standards - U.S. Federal Standard 209 - was first published in 1963,more than 300 normative documents, guidelines or recommended practices on contamination control topics have been published all over the world. Without any doubt they contain valuable advice on many important subjccts.

However, the sheer number of documents and the fact that they have been prepared on a national rather than an international level creates a very unsatisfactory situation in a field as international as cleanroom technology: microelectronics, the pharmaceutical and medical device industries, the emerging nanotechnologies and all the other leading application areas of contamination and biocontamination control technology act and operate globally. The same applies to many of their suppliers of design, testing and qualification services, of cleanroom components and systems as well as of cleanroom disposables - and to all the other industries serving the field of cleanroom technology. A need for international harmonisation was clearly apparent.

In 1993 ISO decided to step in and work on a family of ten globally applicable standards for ***Cleanrooms and Associated Controlled Environments***.

The first ISO standard on cleanrooms was published (June 1999) as 14644-1 '*Classification of Air Cleanliness*'; and the second was issued as an International Standard in September 2000 as 14644-2 '*Specifications for testing and monitoring to prove continued compliance to ISO 14644-1*'. The remaining

Table 2.1: ISO 14644-1 airborne particulate cleanliness classes for cleanrooms and clean zones.

Classification Number (N)	Maximum concentration limits (particles/m^3 of air) for particles equal to and larger than the considered sizes shown below					
	0.1µm	0.2µm	0.3µm	0.5µm	1µm	5.0µm
ISO 1	10	2				
ISO 2	100	24	10	4		
ISO 3	1 000	237	102	35	8	
ISO 4	10 000	2 370	1 020	352	83	
ISO 5	100 000	23 700	10 200	3 520	832	29
ISO 6	1 000 000	237 000	102 000	35 200	8 320	293
ISO 7				352 000	83 200	2 930
ISO 8				3 520 000	832 000	29 300
ISO 9				35 200 000	8 320 000	293 000

eight are in various stages of development, and as of January 2003, yet to be released.

Shown in Table 2.1 is the classification that has been adopted.

The new ISO air cleanliness classification scheme is based on the formula:

$$Cn = 10^{N} (0,1/D)^{2.08} \quad .....(1)$$

Where

Cn = Maximum number concentration of particles per m^3 with diameter equal to or larger than the considered particle diameter, rounded to the nearest whole number, using no more than three significant digits

N = ISO classification number

D = Considered particle diameter in μ m

0,1 = a constant with the dimension μ m

Note: Uncertainties related to the measurement process require that concentration data with no more than three significant figures be used in determining the classification level.

With the selection of 0,1 μm as the reference particle diameter for air cleanliness classification a very straightforward denomination scheme results, thus overcoming elegantly the principal drawback of the metric air cleanliness classes according to U.S. Federal Standard 209E. Simple, single-digit class denominations now correspond with the traditional classes of said standard: ISO *5,* for example, replaces Class 100, and ISO 8 substitutes Class 100 000.

The exponent 2,08 of the correlation between particle concentration and particle diameter ensures the best possible co-incidence with the particle concentrations according to U.S. Federal Standard 209E at that standard's reference particle diameter of 0,5 μm. Thus, a harmonious connection to previous generations of standards is assured.

Determinations for Micro and Macro Particles

In some situations, typically related to specific process requirements, alternative levels of air cleanliness may have to be specified outside the size range of particles applicable to classification. Descriptors have been introduced for coping with such situations as follows:

- the *U descriptor* for ultrafine particles below 0,1 μ m;
- the *M descriptor* for particles above 5 μ m

The U descriptor is expressed in the format :

"(x : y)" .....(2)

where :

x = the maximum permitted concentration of ultrafine particles, expressed as the number of ultrafine particles per m^3 of air

y = the lower detection limit, i.e. the particle size in m m at which the applicable discrete particle counter - for example, a condensation nucleus counter - is capable of detecting such particles with 50 % counting efficiency

The M descriptor is expressed in the format :

"M (a;b);c" .....(3)

where :

a = the maximum permitted concentration of macroparticles, expressed as the number of macroparticles per $m^3$of air

b = the equivalent diameter (or diameters) associated with the specified method for measuring macroparticles

c = the specified method for measuring macroparticles

The concept of the U descriptor is not new - it already forms part of U.S. Federal Standard 209E. On the other hand, the concept of the M descriptor is new. In determining M descriptors, the difficulties of sampling and assessing large particles has to be taken into consideration as well as the fact that large particles are normally process -generated. For these reasons the identification of the sampling device and evaluation procedure should be addressed on an application-specific basis. Factors such as the density, shape, volume and aerodynamic behaviour of the particles need to be taken into account. For describing for instance, an airborne macroparticle concentration of 1000 particles/m^3 in the particle size range of 10 to 20μ m using a cascade impactor for sampling and a microscopic sizing and counting procedure for evaluation, the designation would be :

"M (1 000; 10-20 μ m) : cascade impactor followed by microscopic sizing and counting"

Under certain circumstances it may be necessary, to put special emphasis on specific components of the total airborne particle population, such as fibres. Fibres for instance, may be accounted for by supplementing the M descriptor with a separate descriptor for fibres, having the format "Mfibre (a;b); c".

Cleanroom Testing to prove continued Compliance

At periodic intervals, cleanroom systems should be subjected to a formal requalification procedure. The rules are established in another document of the ISO series of cleanroom technology standards: ISO 14644-2.

Unlike the earlier years where specific values were specified for critical parameters (for example, Air Velocity for Laminar Airflow should be 100 fpm etc) the current standard leaves fixing and determining parametric values entirely to be decided and mutually agreed by the Buyer and Vendor.

ISO 14644-2 determines the type and frequency of testing required to conform to the standard. Table 2.2 indicates which tests are mandatory and Table 2.3 indicates which tests are optional.

Table 2.2 : Strategic Testing (Required)

Schedule of Mandatory tests to demonstrate continuing compliance

Test Parameter	Class	Maximum Time Interval	Test Procedure
Particle Count Test	<= ISO 5 > ISO 5	6 Months 12 Months	ISO 14644-1 Annex A
Air Pressure Difference	All Classes	12 Months	ISO 14644-1 Annex B5
Airflow	All Classes	12 Months	ISO 14644-1 Annex B4

Special Note :

1. Where the installation is equipped with **facilities for continuous or frequent monitoring** of the airborne particulate concentrations and of the differential pressure between rooms, the maximum time interval for the normative tests may be extended to 24 months.
2. In the context of ISO 14644-2, *frequent* monitoring means that measurements should be updated at specified intervals not exceeding

Table 2.3 : Strategic Testing (Optional)

Schedule of additional optional tests			
Test Parameter	**Class**	**Maximum Time Interval**	**Test Procedure**
Installed Filter Leakage	All Classes	24 Months	ISO 14644-3 Annex B6
Containment Leakage	All Classes	24 Months	ISO 14644-3 Annex B4
Recovery	All Classes	24 Months	ISO 14644-3 Annex B13
Airflow Visualization	All Classes	24 Months	ISO 14644-3 Annex B7

60 minutes during utilisation of the cleanroom, ie. in its operational state.

According to this standard, this requalification should comprise at least the following normative tests:

- verification of the *air cleanliness class;*
- verification of *pressure differences* between rooms;
- a verification of the *air velocity* (for displacement airflow) or of the *airflow rate* (for turbulent air-*flow).*

Other tests may optionally be included in the requalification programme as agreed between customer and supplier such as:

- *a leakage or integrity test* for the HEPA filters of the cleanroom system;
- *a recovery test* for cleanrooms with turbulent airflow;
- *a visualisation of the airflow* in the cleanroom;
- *a containment leakage test* for the cleanroom enclosure, i.e. its walls and ceiling.

The test for demonstrating continued particle count compliance should be performed at intervals not exceeding 6 months for cleanrooms of ISO class 5 and below, and at intervals not exceeding 12 months for cleanrooms of class 6 and above. This maximum interval of 12 months also applies for the other normative compliance tests listed above. Where the installation is equipped with facilities for continuous or frequent monitoring, of the airborne particulate concentrations and of the differential pressure between rooms, the maximum time interval for the normative tests may be extended to 24 months. In the context of ISO 14644-2, frequent monitoring means that measurements should be updated at specified intervals not exceeding 60 minutes during utilisation of the cleanroom. i.e. in its operational state.

What is most baffling, however, is the fact that the standard should catogorise a test as *Optional* and in the same breath specify a schedule indicating the maximum time interval between tests. Perhaps it would have been prudent to leave the frequency of testing to the discretion of the User.

Reporting :

The results from testing cleanrooms for compliance with ISO 14644-1 shall be recorded and submitted as a comprehensive report which shall include the following:

- the name and address of the testing organisation, and the date on which the test was performed;
- the number and date of the standard according to which the test was performed i.e. ISO 14644-1: 199x;
- a clear indication of the physical location of the cleanroom tested (including reference to adjacent areas if necessary), and the indication of the co-ordinates of all sampling locations;
- the specified ISO air cleanliness class, the corresponding occupancy state(s), and the considered particle size(s);
- details of the test method used, comprising also any specific conditions relating to the test, or departures from the test method;
- identification of the test instrument(s) and its (their) current calibration certificate(s);
- the test results, including particle concentration data for all sampling location co-ordinates;
- a statement of compliance or non-compliance with the specified ISO air cleanliness class.

An important factor here would be evidence from the Testing Organisation that they are deputing personnel who are qualified to carry out the tests.

Table 2.4 : Comparison of International Standards post ISO

Country and standard						
U.S.A. 209D	U.S.A. 209E	Britain BS 5295	Australia AS 1386	France AFNOR NFX 44-101	Germany VDI 2083	ISO
Date of current issue						
1988	1992	1989	1989	1981	1990	1999
1	M1.5	C	0.035	-	1	3
10	M2.5	D	0.35	-	2	4
100	M3.5	E or F	3.5	4 000	3	5
1 000	M4.5	G or H	35	-	4	6
10 000	M5.5	J	350	400 000	5	7
100 000	M6.5	K	3500	4 000 000	6	8

Very obviously the needs of the pharmaceutical and biotech sectors have not been satisfactorily met by the ISO efforts, which explains the release of guidelines by the MCA, USFDA and WHO in 2002, where parameters and guidelines are more definitive.

Pharmaceutical Cleanroom Classification

EU GGMP 2002

The standards currently prevailing in Europe first came into operation on the 1st of January 1997. This has been retained in the December 2002 release of the EU Guide to Good Manufacturing Practice-Manufacture of Sterile Medicinal Products', or popularly known as the Orange Guide.

The following is an extract of the information that is relevant to the design of cleanrooms.

For the manufacture of sterile medicinal products there are normally four grades of clean areas.

Grade A: *The local zone for high risk operations, eg. filling zones, stopper bowls, open ampoules and vials, making aseptic connections. Normally such conditions are provided by a laminar airflow work station. Laminar airflow systems should provide a homogeneous air speed of 0.45 mps +/- 20% (guidance value) at the working position.*

Grade B: *For aseptic preparation and filling, this is the background environment for Grade A zone.*

Grade C and D: *Clean areas for carrying out less critical stages in the manufacture of sterile products.*

The airborne particulate classification for these grades is given in the following table.

Table 2.5 : Air Classification as per EUGGMP 2002

Grade	Maximum permitted number of particles/m3 equal to or above[1]			
	at rest (b)		in operation	
	0,5μm	5μm	0,5μm	5,0μm
A	3,500	0	3,500	0
B(a)	3,500	0	3,50,000	2,000
C(a)	3,50, 000	2,000	3,500,000	20,000
D(a)	3,500,000	20,000	not defined (c)	not defined (c)

Notes :

1. above or below? Above specified size; below specified number

(a) In order to reach the B, C and D air grades, the number of air changes should be related to the size of the room and the equipment and personnel present in the room. The air system should be provided with appropriate filters such as HEPA for grades A, B and C.

(b) The guidance given for the maximum permitted number of particles in the "at rest" condition corresponds approximately to the US Federal Standard 209E and the ISO classifications as follows: grades A and B correspond with class 100, M 3.5, ISO 5; grade C with class 10 000, M 5.5, ISO 7 and grade D with class 100 000, M 6.5, ISO 8.

(c) The requirement and limit for this area will depend on the nature of the operations carried out.

Examples of operations to be carried out in the various grades are given in the table below.

Table 2.6: EUGGMP 2002: Type of operations for Aseptic preparations

Grade	*Examples of operations for terminally sterilised products*
A	*Filling of products, when unusually at risk.*
C	*Preparation of solutions, when unusually at risk. Filling of products.*
D	*Preparation of solutions and components for subsequent filling.*

Grade	*Examples of operations for aseptic preparations*
A	*Aseptic preparation and filling.*
C	*Preparation of solutions to be filtered..*
D	*Handling of components after washing.*

The particulate conditions given in the table for the "at rest" state should be achieved in the unmanned state after a short "clean up" period of 15-20 minutes (guidance value), after completion of operations. The particulate conditions for grade A in operation given in the table should be maintained in the zone immediately surrounding the product whenever the product or open container is exposed to the environment. It is accepted that it may not always be possible to demonstrate conformity with particulate standards at the point of fill when filling is in progress, due to the generation of particles or droplets from the product itself.

The areas should be monitored during operation, in order to control the particulate cleanliness of the various grades. Where aseptic operations are performed monitoring should be frequent using methods such as settle plates, volumetric air and surface sampling (e.g. swabs and contact plates). Sampling methods used in operation should not interfere with zone protection. Results from monitoring should be considered when reviewing batch documentation for finished product release. Surfaces and personnel should be monitored after critical operations. Additional microbiological monitoring is also required outside production operations, e.g. after validation of systems, cleaning and sanitisation.

Table 2.7: EUGGMP 2002: Recommended limits for microbial contamination [a]

GRADE	air sample cfu/m3	settle plates (diam. 90 mm) cfu/4 hours[b]	contact plates (diam.55 mm) cfu/plate	glove print 5 fingers cfu/glove
A	< 1	< 1	< 1	< 1
B	10	5	5	5
C	100	50	25	-
D	200	100	50	-

Notes :

(a) These are average values.

(b) Individual settle plates may be exposed for less than 4 hours.

Appropriate alert and action limits should be set for the results of particulate and microbiological monitoring. If these limits are exceeded operating procedures should prescribe corrective action.

WHO Guidelines

The World Health Organisation has laid down guidelines that are by and large identical to those by MCA (EU GGMP-2002), except for two significant differences: though the "area" classifications are the same, there is no distinction drawn between the environmental conditions "at rest" and "in operation"; only the ambient bioburden is specified.

Table 2.8 Air Classification as per WHO 2002

Grade	Maximum number permitted / m³		
	Particles		Microorganisms
	0,5µm	5µm	
A (LAF)	3,500	0	less than 1
B	3,500	0	5
C	3,50,000	2,000	100
D	3,500,000	20,000	500

Schedule M 2001

Schedule M 2001 differs from both the EUGGMP 2002 as well as WHO 2002 in several respects, the most significant being the specification for Grade B.

Table 2.9 Air Classification as per Schedule M

Grade	Maximum permitted number of particles/m3 equal to or above[1]			
	at rest (b)		in operation	
	0,5μm	5μm	0,5μm	5,0μm
A	3,520	29	3,500	29
B(a)	35,200	293	3,52,000	2,930
C(a)	3,52,000	2,930	35,20,000	29,300
D(a)	35,20,000	29,300	not defined (c)	not defined (c)

Notes:

(a) In order to reach the B, C and D air grades, the number of air changes should be related to the size of the room and the equipment and personnel present in the room. The air system should be provided with appropriate filters such as HEPA for grades A, B and C.

The maximum permitted number of particles in the "at rest" condition shall approximately be as under: Grade A corresponds with class 100, M 3.5, ISO class 5; Grade B with class 1,000, M 4.5, ISO class 6; Grade C with class 10,000, M 5.5, ISO class 7; Grade D with class 100,000, M 6.5, ISO class 8.

(b) The requirement and limit for this area will depend on the nature of the operations carried out.

(c) Type of operations to be carried out in the various grades are given in the following tables.

TABLE 2.10: Type of operations for Aseptic preparations

Grade	Type of operations for Aseptic preparations
A	Aseptic preparation and filling
B	Background room conditions for activities requiring Grade A
C	Preparation of solutions to be filtered
D	Handling of components after washing

TABLE 2.11: Type of operations for Terminally Sterilised Products

Grade	Type of operations for Terminally Sterilised Products
A	Filling of products, when unusually at risk
C	Placement of filling and sealing machines, preparation of solutions, when unusually at risk. Filling of products when unusually at risk
D	Moulding, blowing (pre-forming) operations of plastic containers, preparation of solutions and components for subsequent filling

TABLE 2.12: Recommended limits for microbiological monitoring of clean areas in operation[(a)]

GRADE	air sample cfu/m3	settle plates (diam. 90 mm) cfu/2 hours[(b)]	contact plates (diam.55 mm) cfu/plate	glove points 5 fingers cfu/glove
A	< 1	< 1	< 1	< 1
B	10	5	5	5
C	100	50	25	-
D	200	100	50	-

Notes:

(a) These are average values.

(b) Individual settle plates may be exposed for not less than 2 hours in Grade B, C and D areas

(c) Appropriate action shall be taken if the results of particulate and microbiological monitoring indicates that the counts exceed limits. The SOPs shall contain corrective action.

Table 2.13: Environmental Monitoring

S/N	Test	Frequency
a	Particle monitoring in air	6 monthly
b	HEPA filter integrity testing (smoke testing)	Yearly
c	Air change rates	6 monthly
d	Air pressure differentials	Daily
e	Temperature and Humidity	Daily
f	Microbiological monitoring by settle plates and/ or swabs in aseptic areas	Daily, and at decreased frequency in other areas

USFDA Guideline on Sterile Drug Products Produced by Aseptic Processing, September 2002

This document was first published in 1987 and is currently undergoing extensive revision. Draft guideline released for comment as "Preliminary Concept Paper" essentially carries all the earlier directives, only further refined.

Table 2.14: Air Classifications[a]

Clean Area Classification	> 0.5 um particles/ft^3	> 0.5 um particles/m^3	Microbiological Limit[b] cfu/10 ft^3	cfu/m^3
100	100	3,500	<1[c]	<3[c]
1000	1000	35,000	<2	<7
10,000	10,000	350,000	<5	<18
100,000	100,000	3,500,000	<25	<88

Notes:

[a]*All classifications based on data measured in the vicinity of exposed articles during periods of activity.*

[b]*Alternate microbiological standards may be established where justified by the nature of the operation.*

[c]*Samples from class 100 environments should normally yield no microbiological contaminants.*

Two clean areas are of particular importance to sterile drug product quality: the critical area and the supporting clean areas associated with it.

Critical and support areas of the aseptic processing operation should be classified and supported by microbiological and particulate data obtained during qualification studies. While initial clean room qualification includes some assessment of air quality under as-built and static conditions, the final room or area classification should be derived from data generated under dynamic conditions, i.e., with personnel present, equipment in place, and operations ongoing. The aseptic processing facility monitoring program should assess conformance with specified clean area classifications under dynamic conditions, on a routine basis.

Parameters other than air cleanliness

So far we have focused on specifying the environmental air cleanliness to suit the application on hand. There are, of course, a whole host of other parameters that need to be specified too. Until a decade ago, most "standards" and "guidelines" indicated "acceptance values". Perhaps this led to over-designing. Perhaps this also led to designs that were inappropriate for the task because the reference documents were silent about some parameter crucial for the application. Thc trcnd today is to offer the Buyer and Vendor adequate latitude in terms of including only those parameters that are relevant, and setting "acceptance" values for the selected parameters, so that they may then work together and produce a facility "fit for use" - neither over-designed, nor under-designed.

Values mentioned in reference documents are often interpreted as inflexible and binding, even if those who authored them did not intend them to be treated so. Many documents today take the extra precaution to clearly mention in parenthesis that the figure given is "guidance value", or "indicative", "illustrative" and not to be interpreted as "mandatory" or "definitive". Despite this cautionary note, I find experts quoting these figures as though they were, indeed, the target values. And once the opinion leader speaks, the rest accept his view as the ultimate interpretation. For example, the Orange Guide states: "Laminar air flow systems should provide a homogeneous air speed of 0.45 m/s +/- 20% (guidance value) at the working position" or "The particulate conditions given for the `at rest' state should be achieved in the unmanned state after a short `clean up' period of 15 - 20 minutes (guidance value), after completion of operations". I have met experts quoting the Orange Guide as though it *mandated* air velocity of 0.45 mps at the work position, and others who interpret the latter statement to mean that any excursion in particulate limits shall be restored to normal within a maximum time interval of 20 minutes.

My interpretation is different. Judging by the spirit in which the entire document has been authored, I am inclined to believe that those who wrote knew very well that terms like "laminar air flow" are obsolete, yet chose to deploy them because they recognised that the words have gathered a denotation and connotation over the decades that best describes the environmental conditions they advocate. They may have said, instead: "sub-turbulent air flow, predominantly unidirectional and with minimum of eddiesat, at the working position". Perhaps they feared that such expressions would confuse more than enlighten. And having exercised the "safe" option, they clarified by mentioning air speeds as has always been defined and understood in the industry to represent LAF. Having done that, they hastened to further clarify that the values mentioned ought not be taken as "definitive" and added the parenthesis. All this amply vindicates my contention that the authors of the current breed of ISO standards demonstrate their wisdom and maturity by pointedly remaining silent, only to avoid such avoidable misinterpretations.

On the other hand, most Buyers, not always being specialists in every detail of project management, find their task of drawing up their Design Qualification documents and setting the criteria for acceptance much easier once they are given clear, irrefutable, measurable acceptance values from an independent, authoritative source. In the absence of such a reference, they are driven to lean heavily on values the Vendors are ever willing to furnish. And when you ask two vendors, it is not uncommon to find two different sets of values!

ISO 14644-4, Cleanrooms and Associated Controlled Environments, Part 4: *Design, construction and start-up*, lists almost every conceivable parameter that may apply, and urges the Buyer and Vendor to identify which are to be included and which are to be ignored, and then go about mutually agreeing to the target values for each.

For those of you who still want some ball park figure to work with, I am reproducing in Table 2.15 values, where mentioned in IES-RP-CC-006, and references for the test methods prescribed. Please use these judiciously.

Norms, methods and techniques that have been established and proven to constitute Good Manufacturing Practice are codified as a *standard* for others to refer and freely drew upon. Standards must therefore be viewed as a *reflection* of Industry norms, historical documents that prescribe the *lowest common denominator* for minimal compliance requirements. The benchmarks in a standard represent the floor, rather than the ceiling. By this token, your specifications should be drawn to *better* compendial limits, not just *meet* them. Because it is quite probable that no sooner the ink dries on the first standard,

Table 2.15: Indicative Acceptance Values

Parameter	References	Unidirectional	Turbulent	Mixed	Acceptance	
					Rooms	LF Devices
Main Air Supply Volume	ACMA 203				MA	N/A
Make up Air Supply Volume	ACMA 203				MA	N/A
Reserve Capacity of Main AHU	ACMA 203				MA	N/A
Air volume & uniformity	ISO 14644-3	1,2,3	1,2,3	1,2,3	5%	10%
Air velocity & uniformity	ISO 14644-3	1,2,3	O	O	5%	24 - 30 m/min
Airflow visualisation	ISO 14644-3				MA	MA
Airflow direction	ISO 14644-3				MA	MA
Installed Filter Leak	ISO 14644-3	1,2	1,2	1,2	0.01%	0.01%
Particle Count	ISO 14644-3	1,2,3	1,2,3	1,2,3	<UCL	MA
Ultrafines Count	ISO 14644-3				MA	MA
Macro-Particles Count	ISO 14644-3				MA	N/A
Microbial Count	MCA/WHO/M				MA	MA
Pressurisation	ISO 14644-3	1,2,3	1,2,3	1,2,3	MA	N/A
Parallelism[a]	ISO 14644-3	1,2	-	O (1,2 only)	14°	14°
Integrity/Containment Leak	ISO 14644-3	1,2	1,2	1,2	$< 10^{-3}$	0.01%
Induction/Back streaming	IES-RP-CC-002/6				$< 10^{-3}$	Nil
Recovery	ISO 14644-3	N/A	1,2	1,2	MA	N/A
Particle Fallout/Deposition	ISO 14644-3	1,2,3	1,2,3	1,2,3	MA	N/A
Lighting Level	IES-RP-CC-002/6	1,O (2,3)	1,O (2,3)	1,O (2,3)	MA	800 lumens/m^2
Electrostatic & Ion Generator	ISO 14644-3				MA	MA
Noise Level	IES-RP-CC-002/6	1,2	1,2	1,2	MA	< 67 dbA
Temperature uniformity	ISO 14644-3	1,2,3	1,2,3	1,2,3	(1 - 0.05 °C)	Rise < 5.6 °C
Moisture uniformity	ISO 14644-3	O	O	O	MA	N/A
Vibration	IES-RP-CC-002/6	O	O	O	MA	< 5μ rms at 10 - 200Hz

new frontiers are crossed and manufacturing technology nudges further, rendering the current standard obsolete, necessitating revision to stay in tune with current Good Manufacturing Practice. And you will find yourself ever running only to find yourself in the same place.

Key to Table 2.15

O	Test optional depending on requirements
1	Test suited to as-built phase
2	Test suited to at-rest phase
3	Test suited to operating phase
a	Entry and exit planes to be at least 900 mm apart, or as MA
N/A	Not applicable
MA	As mutually agreed between buyer & seller

Special requirements for ISO Class 3 cleanroom

Air quality	:	Total hydrocarbons < 1 ppm; Na < 0.1 μ g/m^3
Fresh air intake	:	0.5 m^3/min per sqm of cleanroom floor area
Vibration	:	< 0.1μ (building); < 0.01μ (equipment) rms
Noise	:	< 55 dbA
Temperature var	:	< 0.1 °C
Humidity	:	< 2%
Magnetic field var	:	< 1 mG
Static charge	:	< 50 V

3 Elements of Cleanroom Design Engineering

Design of clean spaces or cleanrooms encompasses much more than the traditional control of temperature, humidity and make-up air to keep the environment acceptably "fresh". Other parameters that must be factored into the design include control of suspended particulates, both viable and non-viable, vapours and fumes, pressure gradients, airflow velocities and airflow patterns, cross-contamination, noise, vibration, and electrostatic discharge. Another distinctive characteristic is the high level of control called for in the design, customising to suit the equipment and layout within the clean shell.

HVAC for cleanrooms

While there are as many HVAC designs as designers, the mark of a good design lies in its ability to control these parameters with due regard to industrial engineering, energy conservation and safety aspects at reasonable installation, operation and maintenance costs.

Good Design Practice requires careful assessment of the facility requirements, and involvement at the conceptual stage itself knowledgeable and experienced representatives from design, construction, commissioning, qualification, operations, production and maintenance. Which is one motivation behind the clause "as agreed between Buyer and Vendor" that the ISO documents are so full of. It is particularly important to set target values, variance limits and the criteria for acceptance for each parameter.

A design that considers such maintainability concerns as accessibility for cleaning, testing and repairs; frequency of maintenance; and availability of spare parts as important requirements is likely to prove much more reliable in operation. Failure can compromise the process.

In today's document driven world, the first step is in creating a Qualification Plan for HVAC, which includes:

1. A functional description of what the system will do
2. Maps of room pressures, airflow diagrams, and cleanliness zones served by each air handler
3. A list of critical components to be qualified
4. A list of the User's procedures that must be followed for the qualification of equipment and systems that affect critical variables
5. A list of qualification procedures (DQ/IQ/OQ/PQ protocols) that must be written specially for the project
6. A list of needed commissioning equipment
7. The procedure (or criteria)for approval and acceptance

HVAC is too complex a subject, specially where it concerns cleanrooms, to be glossed over in a chapter of a book such as this one. It merits a book, or a handbook, by itself. And an excellent reference book available is the one published by ASHRAE, where the design approach is discussed with an application bias. I shall restrict myself to merely highlighting the HVAC components, and throw in some tips that the designers may find useful.

Understanding HVAC Components

High side: *Air tempering system*		**Low side: *Air distribution system***	
Refrigeration system	Compressor	Air Handling Unit	Filters
Condensor	Chiller	Booster blowers	Supply air ducts
Evaporator	Heat exchanger	Return air ducting	Fresh air system
Humidifier	Mixing valves	Exhaust air system	

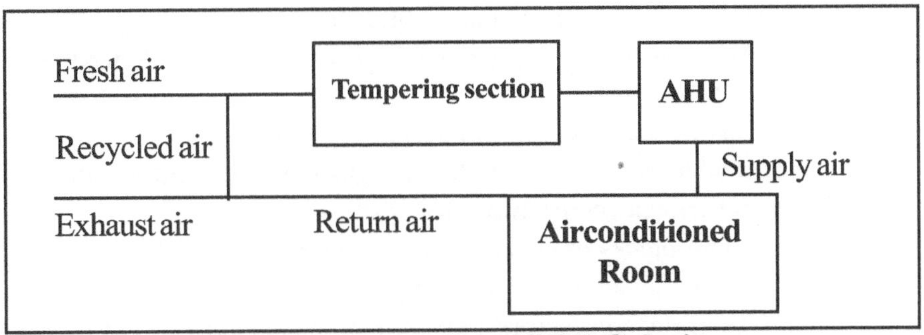

Fig. 3.1: Conventional HVAC design

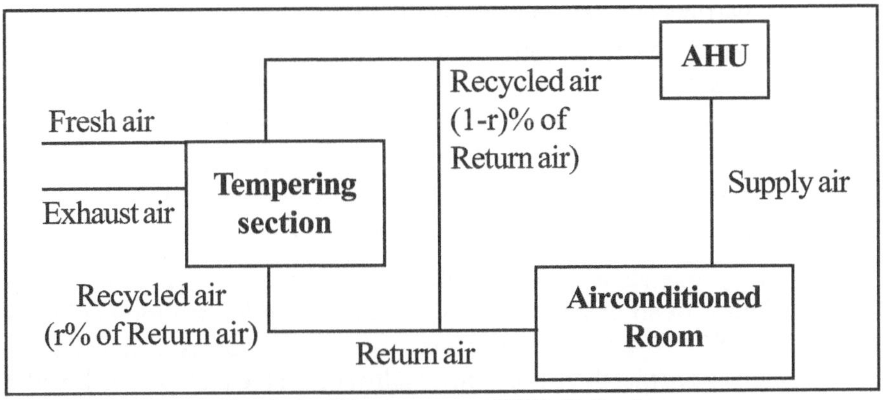

Fig. 3.2:Cleanroom HVAC design

Tips for Cleanroom HVAC Design

Temperature Control

1. Identify the control zones
2. Try restrict size of control zones: 14'-16' W x 20' - 40' L
3. For more stringent control, reduce size further
4. Try distributing process heat generation evenly
5. Ensure proper insulation of structure
6. Ensure proper treatment of fresh/ make-up air
7. Effectively balance air quantities in areas needing exhaust
8. Ensure proper cooling systems for equipment
9. Provide airlocks and change rooms

Noise/Vibration Control

1. Select quiet equipment
2. Use sound absorbing materials on ducts and wherever else permissible
3. Design ducts and fittings for low turbulence

4. Locate high velocity ducts in non-critical areas
5. Isolate pipes, ducts and sound plenums from structure with neoprene or spring hangers
6. Select fans for minimum sound power
7. Use duct silencers and sound plenums in supply and return ducts
8. Locate equipment rooms away from critical areas
9. Use masonry blocks or concrete for equipment room walls and floor
10. Balance rotating and reciprocating equipment
11. Install flexible connectors between pipes, ducts and vibrating equipment
12. Use barriers and covers to interrupt noise paths
13. Design and install duct attenuation to match transmission loss through walls between rooms
14. Extend partition to ceiling slab and tightly seal all around
15. Seal all pipe, conduit, duct and other penetrations through partition
16. Mount all machines on properly designed vibration isolators
17. Design mechanical equipment for dynamic loads

Misconceptions abound on the subject of optimal air change rate for a prescribed class of air cleanliness. HVAC convention for comfort cooling is in the range of 2 to 6 air changes per hour. But when it comes to air cleaning, not many are aware that there is no universally applicable thumb rule. Besides not many differentiate between the air change rate and the *effective dilution rate,* which takes into account the additional clean down caused by the LAF work stations in the room. Since this varies from facility to facility, the optimal air change rate as well as effective dilution rate must be worked out case by case. The table below is purely indicative.

Table 3.1: Industry thumb rules

ISO Class	Controls	Air Velocity at table level (fpm)	Air Change Rate (per hour)	HEPA Coverage as % of Ceiling
1	Stringent	70 - 130	>750	100
2	Stringent	70 - 130	>750	100
3	Stringent	70 - 130	>750	100
4	Stringent	70 - 110	500 - 600	100
5	Stringent	70 - 90	150 - 400	100
6	Intermediate	25 - 40	60 - 100	33 - 40
7	Intermediate	10 - 15	25 - 40	10 - 15
8	Less Stringent	3 - 5	10 - 15	5 - 10

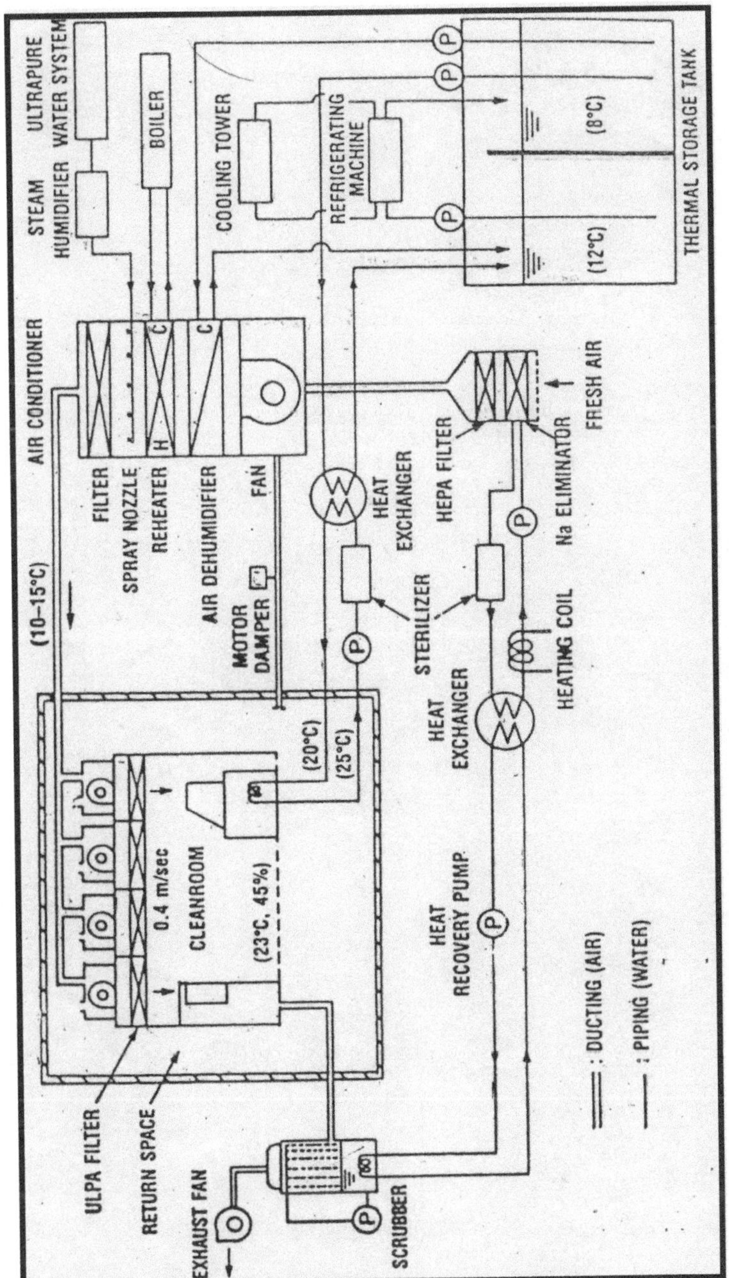

Fig. 3.3: HVAC schematic for a typical cleanroom airconditioning system

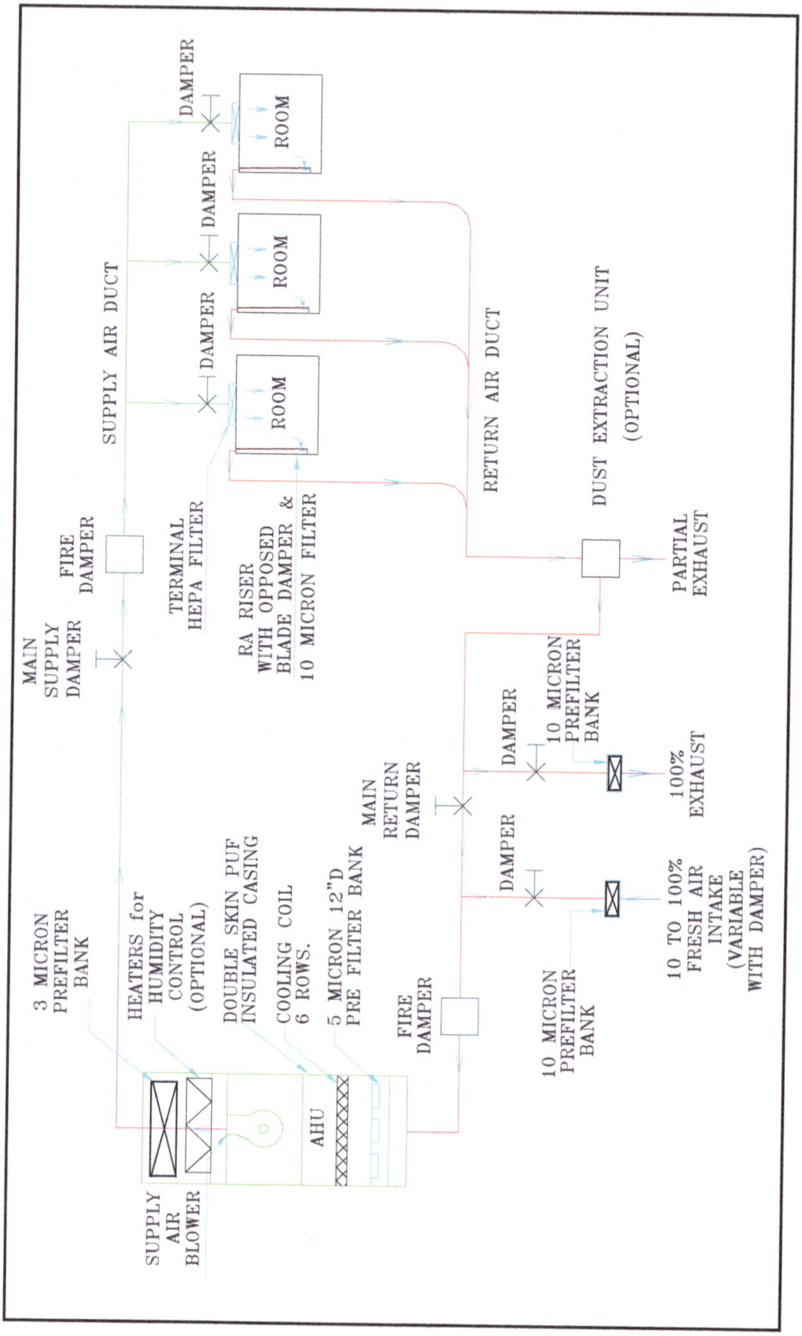

Fig. 3.4: HVAC schematic for cleanroom: recycled air

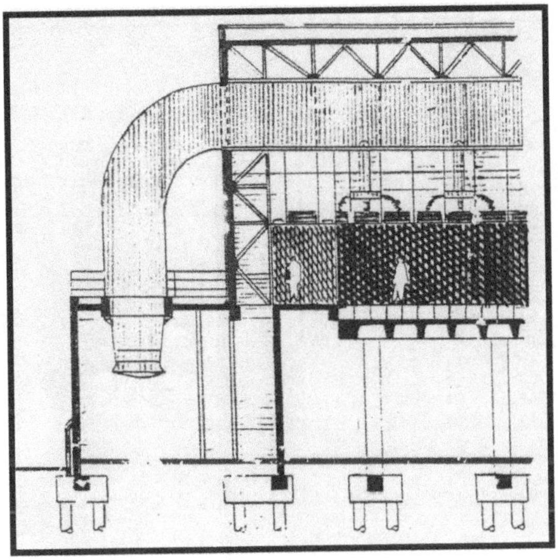

Fig. 3.5: Overhang structure for low vibration in Wafer Fabs

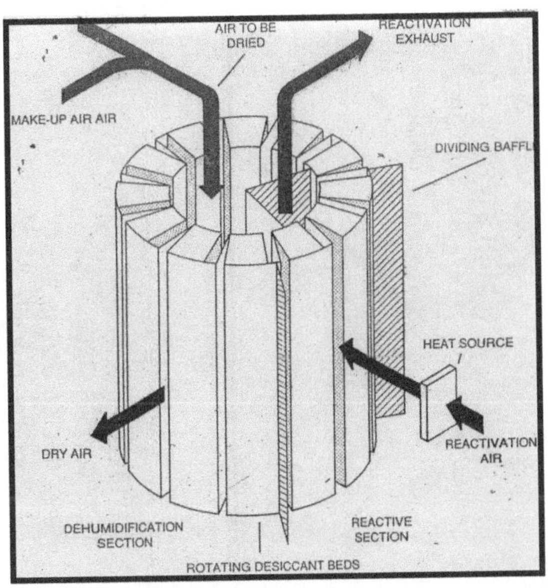

Fig. 3.6: Cleanroom Dehumidification System

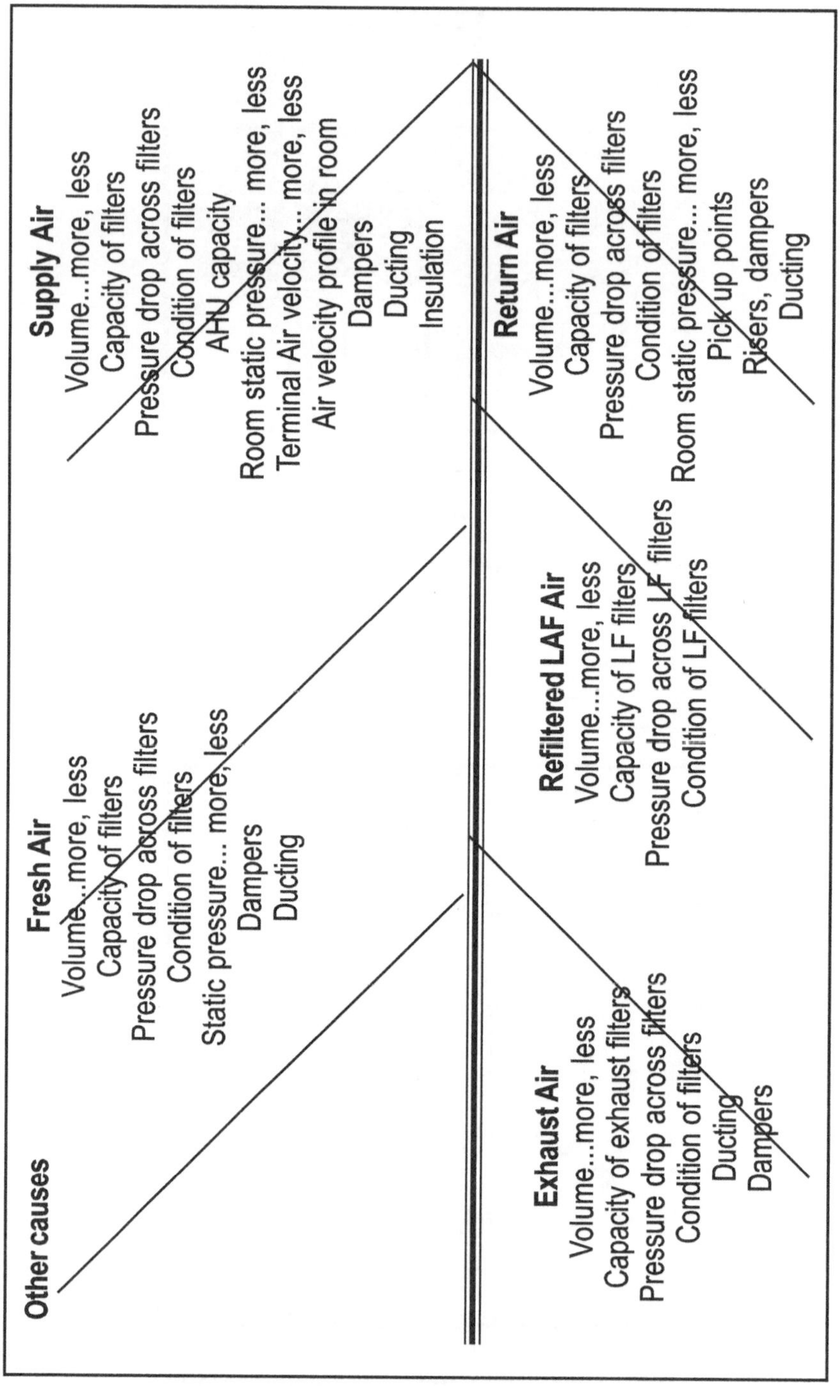

Fig. 3.7: Fish Bone Diagram: Air Management - Cause & Effect

Air filtration and distribution

Air filtration and distribution forms the core of airborne contamination control. It also represents a major investment block in the project.

Early designs favoured massive air handling units with large banks packed with air filters located remote from the cleanroom. This is understandable, since at that time the cleanroom was seen as a natural extension of HVAC engineering, and the system bore their unmistakable signature.

By the time the filtered air reached the work space it had lost much of its purity. The Users began interacting, and together they evolved a configuration that brought final filtration as close to the point of use as possible, and returned the air from floor level for improved particle scavenging , a departure from convention which relied on convective forces to propel warm air upwards. The emphasis had shifted from *tempering* the air to *cleansing* thc air.

Terminal filters in the ceiling supplying clean air into the room from scattered locations is a configuration known as *turbulent flow* cleanroom. The air that emanates from the filter moves downwards. In the absence of constraining panels, it also moves laterally and diffuses. The velocity gradients at point of entry may be compared with the air jet model, where Bernoulli venturi effects are pronounced and produce vortices, eddies and induced air currents. As a consequence, the airflow rate, air velocity and suspended contaminant density profiles across the cross-section of the room varies sinusoidally from one filter location to the next. There are a significant number of pockets either stagnant or turbulent. These zones can be identified using visualisation techniques that employ fogs, smoke or bubbles whose densities are the same as the ambient air.

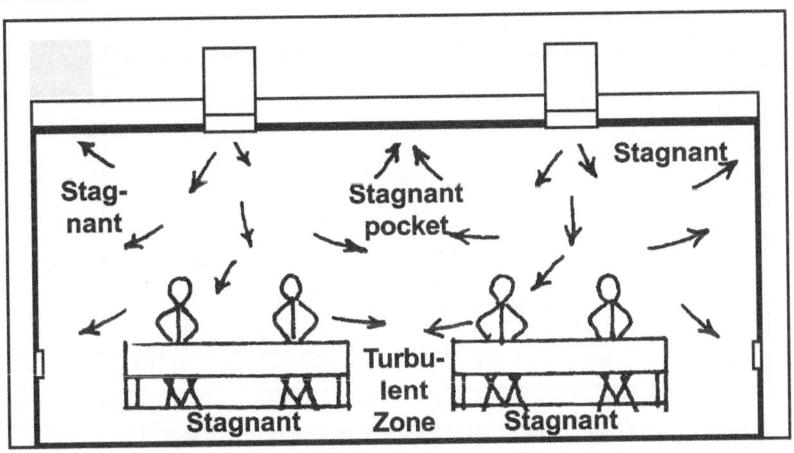

Fig. 3.8: Turbulent airflow cleanroom

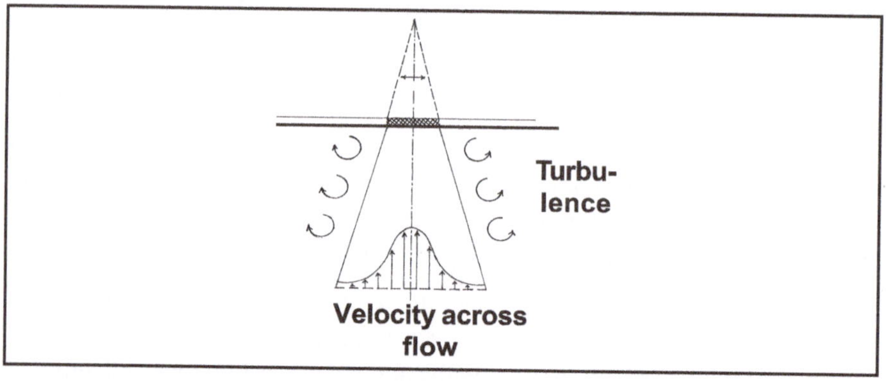

Fig. 3.9: Approximate flow profile of air exiting from terminally mounted HEPA filter

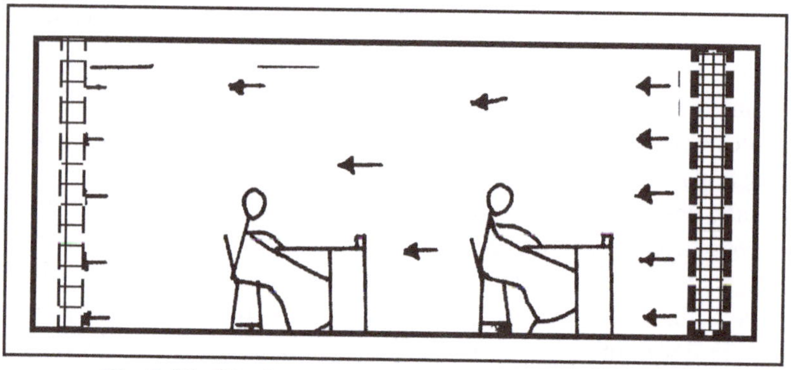

Fig 3.10: Horizontal laminar airflow cleanroom

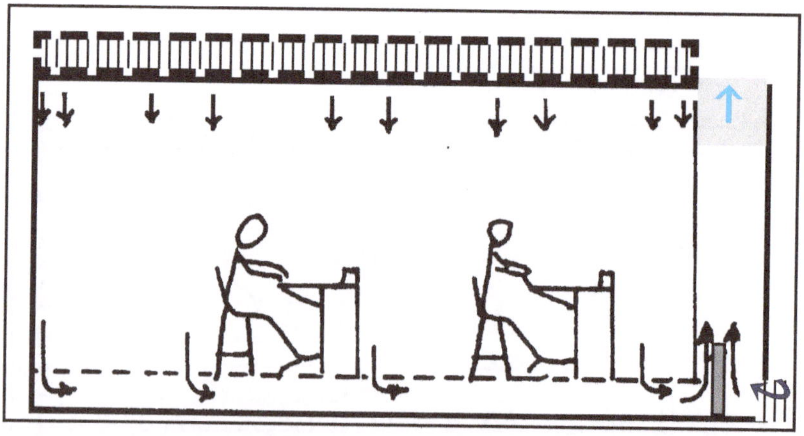

Fig. 311: Vertical laminar downflow cleanroom with perforated floor

Substantial improvement is attained when the entire ceiling forms a near-monolithic matrix of juxtaposed filters. This is the *mixed flow* cleanroom. Parametric profiles are more uniform, but vortices and stagnant pockets are not eliminated altogether, since air diverges from the centre of the room towards the periphery of the floor where the return air chases are located.

Turbulence and stagnation hinder the clean down process. We can not aspire for environment air cleanliness much beyond Class 1000 with the mixed flow model, or Class 10,000 with the turbulent flow model. As the need for more stringent environmental air cleanliness rose, the mixed flow concept was further refined to avoid divergence of the air stream at every plane, and the return was directed to a raised perforated floor, beneath which ran the return air chases. Air velocity was controlled and retained in the unidirectional flow range. As a result, suspended contaminants were flushed out by pistons of clean air, with the four walls serving as flow directing and constraining panels. This configuration is the *vertical laminar down flow* cleanroom or Vertical LAF clean tunnel. A variation embracing the same design principles is the *horizontal laminar airflow* cleanroom or the horizontal LAF clean tunnel, where clean air enters the room from a filtered wall and exits from the opposite facing wall, moving clean air 'laterally' like a piston. Over the past decade, the term "laminar flow" has been replaced by "Unidirectional flow". Parametric profiles are highly consistent and uniform across the length and breadth of the room, with variations, if any, extremely localised and directly traceable to some contaminant generating activity at, or peculiar to, that location.

The emphasis in today's world is increasingly on flexibility, and the ability to modify, upgrade and adapt to changing technologies and needs. The cleanroom configurations we have discussed so far are difficult to modify, and impossible to relocate.

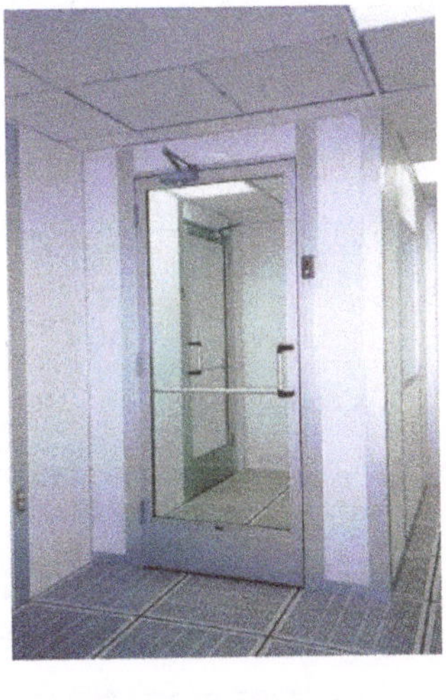

Fig 3.12: Modular prefabricated cleanroom

Over the past decade Users have increasingly favoured prefabricated clean rooms. A typical installation takes a crew of less than five persons less than two weeks to commission a facility of 2000 sq ft, starting from scratch. One can imagine the benefits of the drastic reduction in lead time and the bother of coordinating with multiple external subcontract agencies. As growth opportunities thin out professionals at

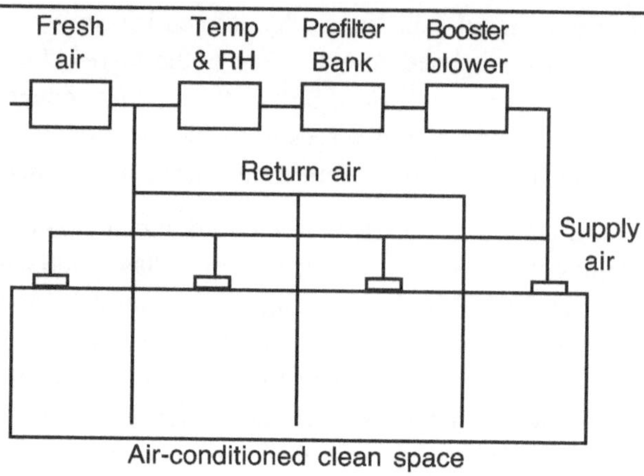

Air-conditioning system with booster blower, prefilters mounted in a bank on the suction side of blower. Air is then ducted into the room through terminal HEPA filters. Return air is drawn from floor level through tapered risers.

Fig 3.13: Turbulent airflow with low-level return air scavenging

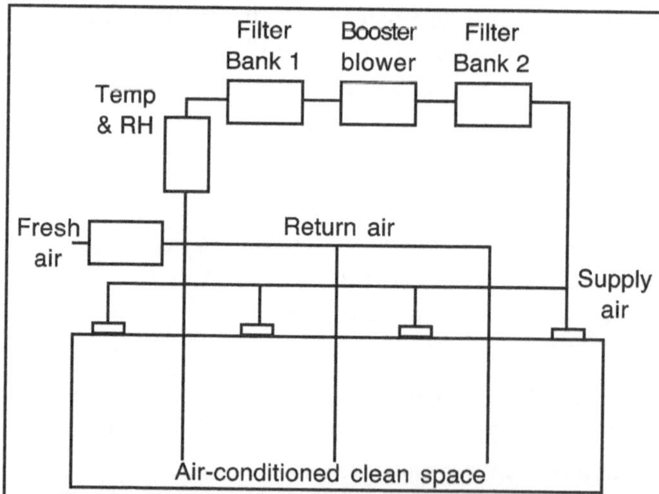

Air-conditioning system with booster blower, two filter banks, one comprising prefilters on the suction side, and another, which may be pre- or HEPAs, on the delivery side, Air is then ducted into the room through terminal HEPA filters . Return air is drawn from floor level through tapered risers.

Fig 3.14: Turbulent airflow as above, but with additional filtration

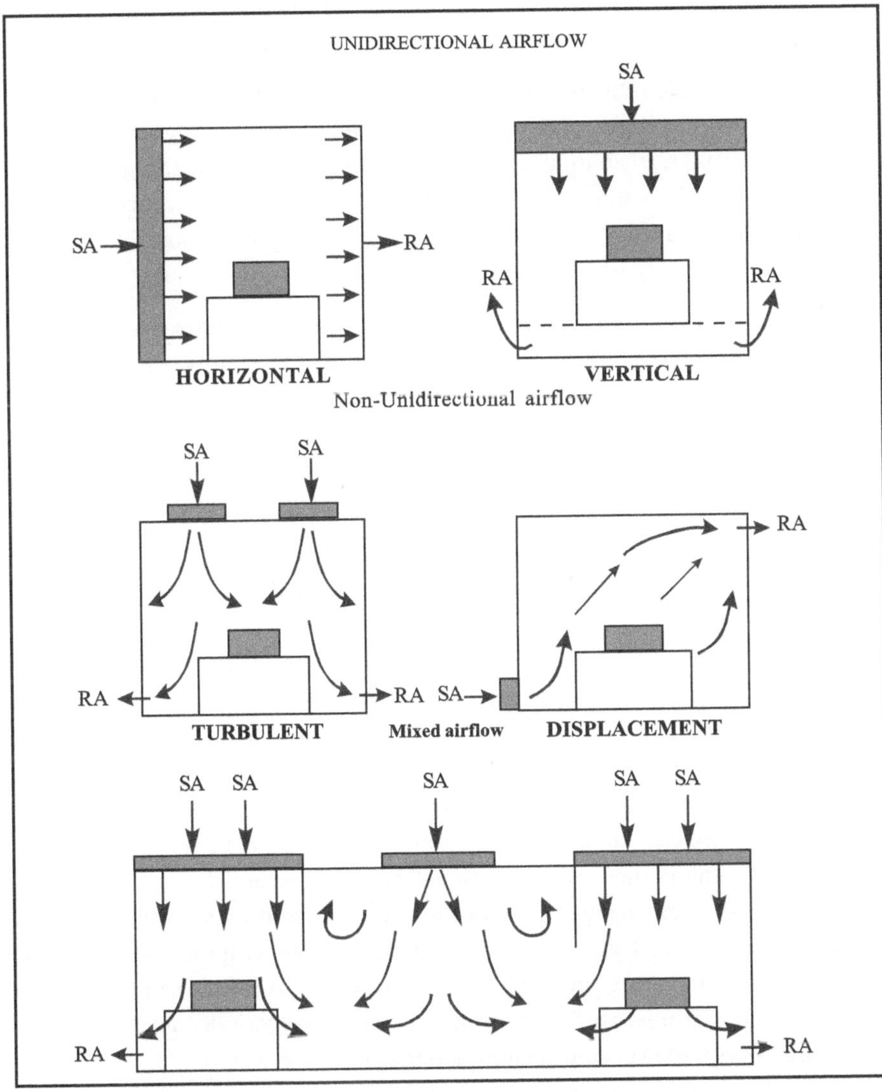

Fig. 3.15: Airflow patterns in cleanrooms described in ISO 14644-4

Note : SA is supply air ; RA is return air

every level, many users find this approach to cleanroom construction makes eminent sense, since it does not call for high level in-house skills. What is most appealing, however, is that the facility can be easily relocated at a fraction of the original cost, or be enlarged, upgraded, or downsized at will.

The prefabricated cleanroom comes with a smooth, cleanable panelised shell, optional raised perforated tiled floor, return air ducting and plenum, adjustment dampers, in-built utilities and a ceiling complete with lights. Since all equipment and ancillaries can be mounted outside the cleanroom shell in the service chase, access for service, preventive or repair, is possible without breach of the integrity of the facility.

Not every location in the cleanroom may require the same quality of air: some may need more, some less. By adjusting the supply and return air distribution it is possible to grade the cleanroom such that air supply volume is increased in some areas, and reduced in others. This is known as *zoning* the cleanroom. These areas may be physically separated using panels and enclosures, called *hard* separation, or using air velocity gradients, called *soft* separation. Hard separators cause abrupt changes in the air velocity field at the boundary (where the velocity is zero), which in turn creates pressure gradients (Bernoulli effect) that produce turbulence and induce secondary air currents from outside the boundary.

Some prefabricated designs incorporate *smart* components. To cite one example, as dirt accumulates on the filter the blower *automatically* increases its speed of rotation to maintain airflow rates at design levels. Some systems change the airflow rate on need-base supply. For instance, the change room traffic is at its heaviest at start-up and shutdown; at these times the supply to the change rooms is increased; at other times it is reduced. Similarly, the *sleep* feature in some designs switches off the refrigeration system altogether at the end of the shift and cuts down on air supply volume to levels just enough to maintain overpressure, switching back to normal mode before commencement of next shift, sufficiently ahead to restore design conditions. These are energy conserving techniques that must be welcomed.

An important characteristic of any cleanroom design is the *residence* time. How long does a contaminant linger within the environment on an average? By corollary we also determine the *decay* time, and *recovery* time. For example, whenever an aberration occurs, as during an accidental spill or explosion, what is the contaminant density profile on a time scale before normal mode operation is restored.

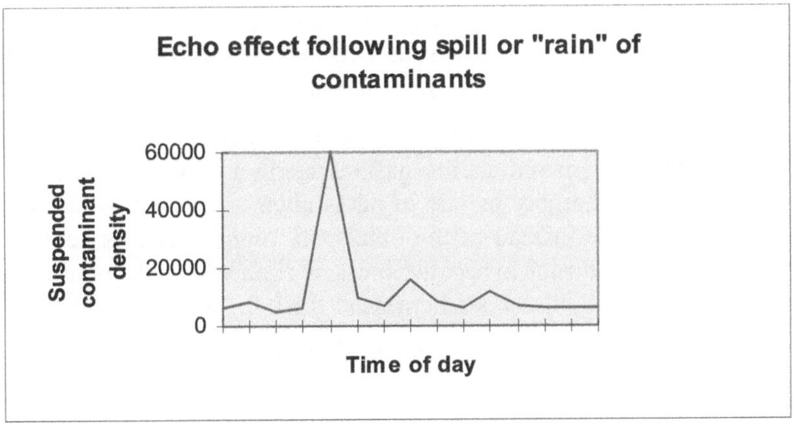

Fig 3.16: Cleanroom recovery

Whenever there is an excursion in the particulate desnsity, like a cloud or shower of contaminants suddenly introduced into or generated within the room, the contaminant peak will be followed by a series of ripple peaks or *echo* effects, each time the *contaminated air volume* returns to the room. Because of refiltration on every cycle, the peak amplitude progressively diminishes.

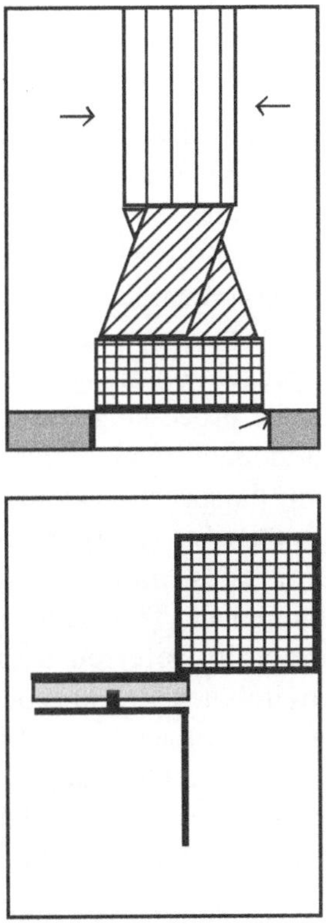

Fig 3.17: HEPA mounting

Mounting a terminal filter is as important as selecting the filter. Terminal filters execution is either box- or cassette-type, where fitting is from over head, or flange type, where fitting is from within the cleanroom. The latter is generally preferred, except where the ceiling is a service mezzanine floor with cutouts for the filter housings, because it is more convenient. But this causes a more serious breach of the environment each time the filter has to be attended to for any reason.

How effectively the filter is seated and sealed depends on the filter housing design, and the arrangements for clamping it in position. All filters feature mounting gaskets, usually closed cell neoprene rubber. But when two flat surfaces are pressed together, more often than not, there is leakage at some point or other. To overcome this inherent deficiency, some designs feature a knife-edge on one of the two surfaces, while the other features the gasket. When clamped down, any unevenness in the two mating surfaces is taken care of by the line contact of the knife-edge as it embeds itself into the gasket.

Yet another ingenious innovation features the *negative pressure* seal. Leaks through ill-fitted filters and ageing gaskets being a perennial problem, this design makes sure that any bypass of air is always directed from the *clean* side to the *dirty* side instead of the other way round. This is achieved by immersing the filter housing in negative pressure connected to the return plenum. The same concept has also been harnessed for LAF work benches.

Current breed of terminal filters installed in higher grade cleanrooms are gasketless, and use a fluid seal such as a petroleum blend or silicone or urethane gel.

The cost of design and construction of clean rooms has risen astronomically over the past decade. Like first cost, the operating costs of a cleanroom have gone up in direct relationship to the cleanliness level of the facility. Additionally, a cleaner facility equates to more restrictive practices, often reducing the efficiency of operations performed.

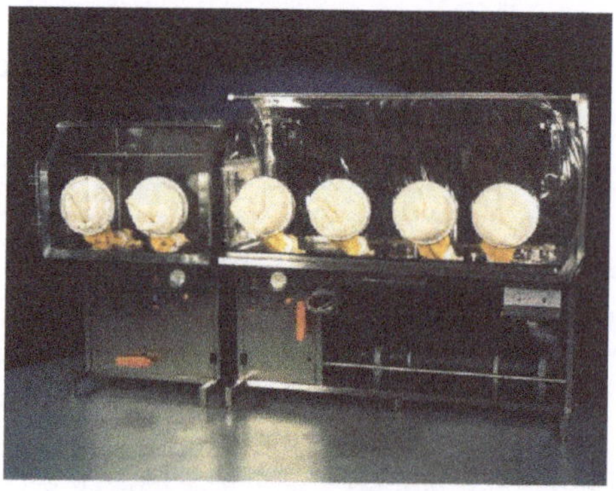

Fig 3.18: Isolators

These trends are increasingly driving cleanroom users and designers to seek alternative solutions. Foremost among those being contemplated is the reduction of clean space to the minimum practical volume, generally related to the processing equipment used in the facility and may encompass only the space containing the critical product, or a larger volume that embraces most or all of the equipment. The reduced volume is generally referred to as a *mini-environment* or a *microenvironment*, depending on the level of size reduction, and the prime concept driving this is *isolation* technology. A mini-environment seeks to exclude people, while encasing the equipment from floor to ceiling; a microenvironment seeks to isolate only the product, leaving out much of the less critical parts of the equipment itself.

Isolation technology is not the construction of boxes over equipment and the ducting of clean air into such boxes. It is a science involving development of clean environments and isolation of those environments from contamination sources, and consists of four basic areas of study:

- √ Identifying the areas that require the cleanest conditions
- √ Developing barriers to prevent migration of contaminants into these environments. These barriers may be *hard, soft*, or *semi-soft* (flexible PVC) or any combination of these.
- √ A system must be devised for safe and facile movement of items not only into and out of the environments, but also from one isolated environment to another.
- √ A methodology to breach these isolated environments without detrimental effects.

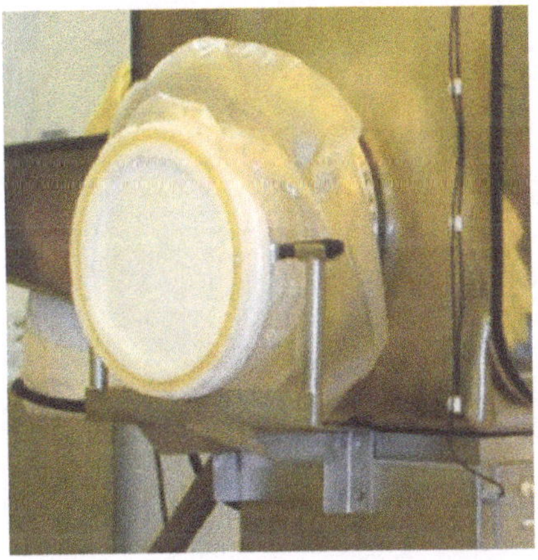

Fig 3.19: Isolator transfer hatch featuring α-β door interlocking

Though mini- and micro-environments featuring isolation technology are referred to in the Orange Guide 2002, the Draft USFDA Guidelines for Aseptic Processing, and a separate ISO Standard is in the pipeline: **ISO 14644-7:** *Cleanrooms and Associated Controlled Environments, Part 7: Separative enclosures (clean air hoods, glove boxes,isolators, minienvironments).* This has already been issued as draft international standard: **DIS 14644-7.**

Having said that, however, it must also be mentioned that the much promised reductions in cost with such facilities has remained unfulfilled, and it is likely to take a while before these emerge as a viable alternative or gain wide spread acceptance, sufficient to obsolete current options.

Cleanroom shell and area layout: points to ponder

- The greater the physical isolation of the product or process from the outside, the easier the task of preventing ingress of suspended contaminants. The manner in which the work area is designed, and the manner in which work is carried out inside have a direct influence on the yield.
- Keep the size as small as possible. The smaller the footprint, the easier it is to manage, maintain and control. Large blocks should, to the extent feasible, be broken and subdivided into smaller homogeneous blocks, leaving just enough scope for expansions in the foreseeable future. Large rooms have uneven parametric profiles.

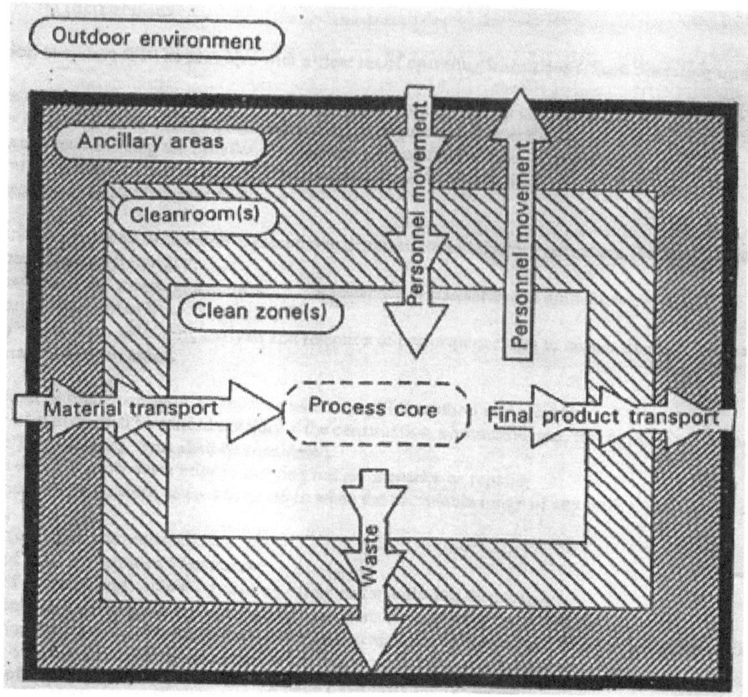

Fig 3.20: Segregation concept described in DIS: ISO 14644-4

- Operations and equipment that do not necessarily have to be inside the cleanroom should be kept out.
- Take into account the natural flow path of the process and dove tail the material and manpower flow paths to be congruent with it. Movements should be minimal, unidirectional, with little or no looping. To & fro movements increase contamination risks.
- Where more than one product is planned for sequential production, check for product compatibility, and cleandown requirements.
- If more than one product is to be produced simultaneously, it is better to have dedicated facilities rather than a shared facility. Cross-contamination is an ever present threat.
- Common entryways may make economic sense; but they do not always make good GMP sense. Check carefully before you decide.
- Incompatible products should not only be isolated physically, but should have dedicated and independent air handling systems. This aspect is often overlooked.

Typical steps in various processes: area layout, equipment layout, and movement of men and materials should be dove-tailed to these steps to ensure congruency and preclude loops and overlaps.

Semicon Wafers
Wafer cleaning
Diffusion
Lithography (etching)
Metallisation
Plasma etch
Laser trim
Bevel lap
Edge polish
Passivation

Semicon Packaging
Wafer dicing
Die attach
Wire bonding
Testing
Curing
Lead frame tip plating
Encapsulation
Post moulding testing & branding

Vaccines
Media preparation
Subculture bacteria
Dilution of bacteria in liquid media
Centrifuge & retain supernatant
0.22micron filtration
Column chromatography
Concentrate toxin protein
Bioassay in rabbit illeal loops
Immunisation

Bio-assay
Sub-culture of bacteria
Sample dilution
Standard dilution
Assay dilution
Media preparation
Media discharge
Volume make-up with water
Sterilisation at 121°C/15 min
Cooling

Fig 3.21: Process flow charts

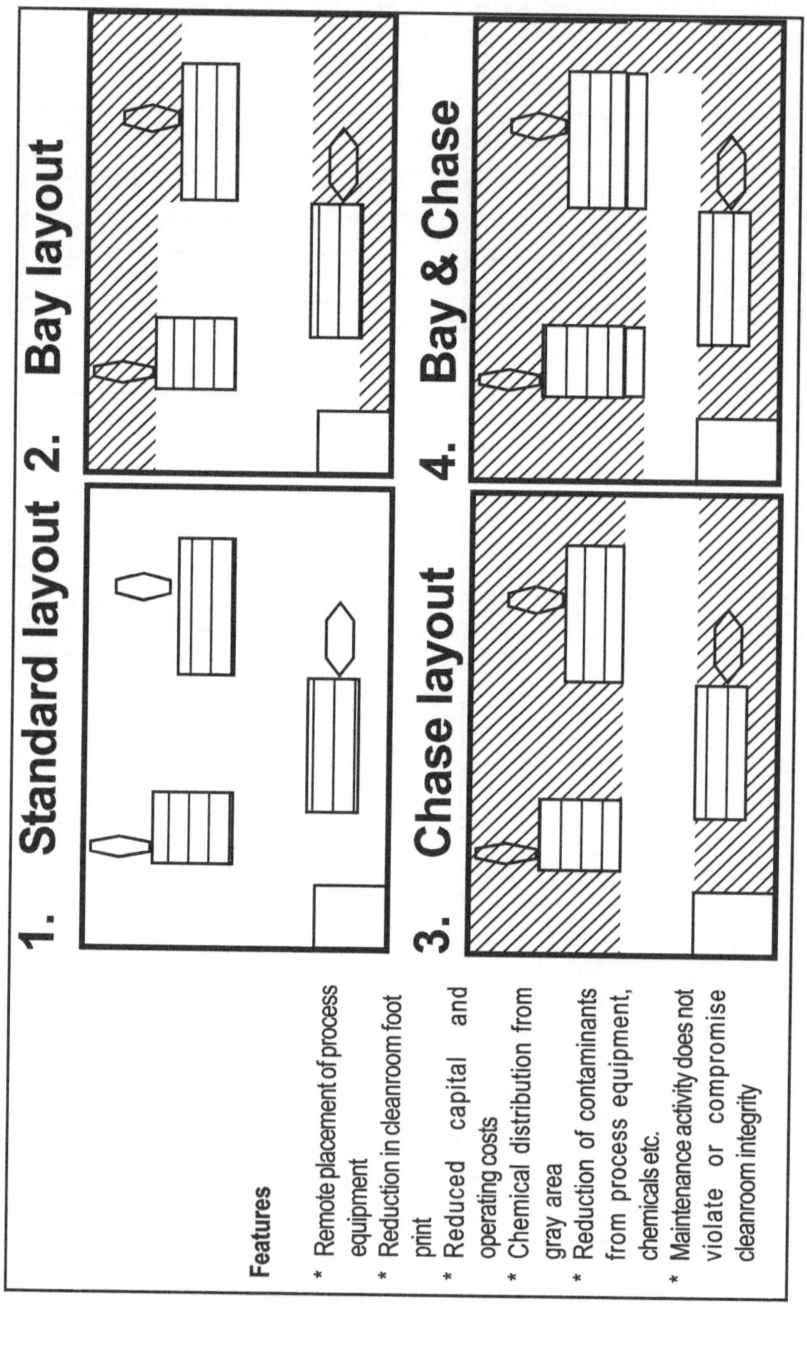

Fig. 3.22: Optimising Area Layout: Progressive minimisation of Footprint

- Operations that generate excessive contaminants like grinding, polishing, powder milling and mixing should be nowhere near the critical zone.
- Keep away from toilets, kitchens and other "wet" areas.
- Sinks and drains should be prohibited in critical zones (Grades A/B) used for aseptic manufacture. In less stringent zones, air breaks should be fitted between the machine or sink and the drains. Floor drains in lower grade cleanrooms should be fitted with traps or water seals to prevent backflow.
- Avoid direct pathways; stagger doorways; build a buffer zone that envelopes the critical zone.
- It is common practice to have doors opening inwards into a room under over-pressure, so that the door seals snugly when shut. This configuration causes ripples inside the critical zone each time someone opens the door to enter or exit. The bellow effect induces an artifact on the differential pressure across terminal filters. The full implication can best be appreciated using air stream visualisation.

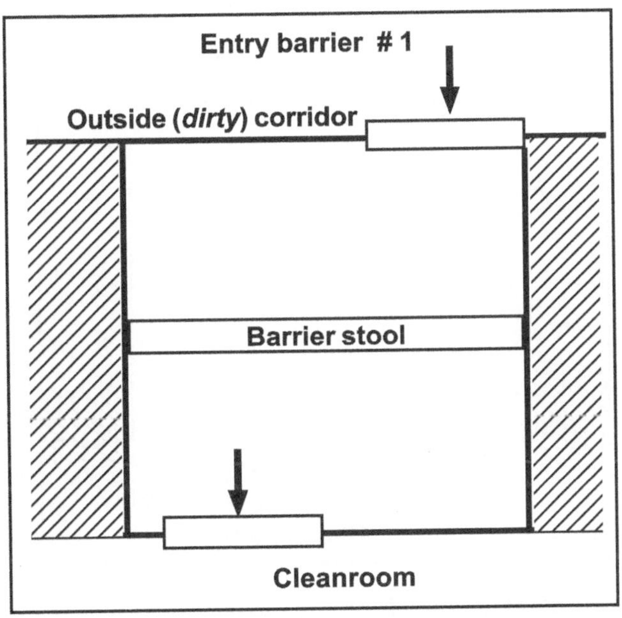

Fig. 3.23: H-barrier for personnel

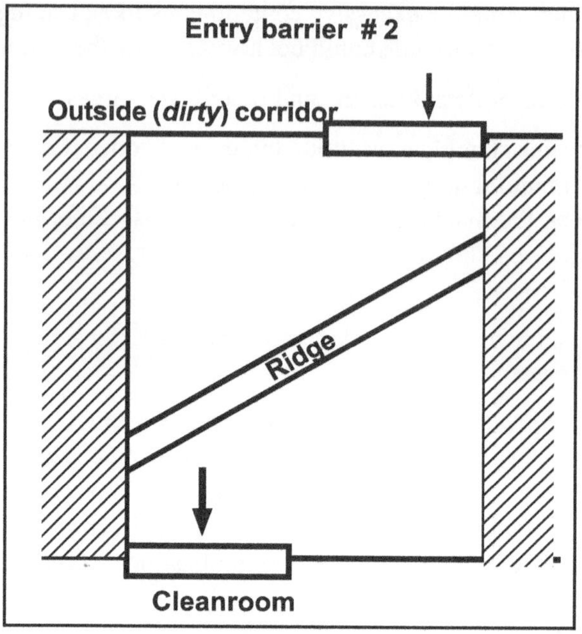

Fig. 3.24: Z-barrier to separate cleanroom side from outside in material entry airlock

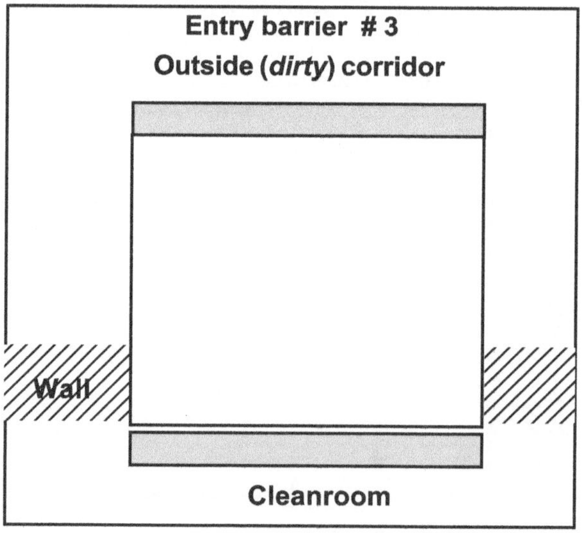

Fig. 3.25: Double-door interlocked pass-through window for transfer of small items

- Airlock doors should not be opened simultaneously. An interlocking system or a visual/audible warning system should be installed to prevent more than one door being opened at the same time.
- Avoid external walls; if not feasible, avoid windows on external wall. Avoid west facing wall.
- Provide for separate entry routes for equipment and materials, and personnel.
- Entry ways for personnel may require subdivisions for male and female operators. Wash and toilet blocks should be located as remotely as possible from the product site.
- Provide H-barrier to demarcate grey zone from black zone.
- Provide for lockers, footwear and garment storage.
- Provide staging area for decontamination of material and equipment prior to entry.
- Provide Z-barrier in anteroom for trolleys, where material brought in may be transferred across the barrier from one trolley to the other. Keep separate trolleys for transporting material exclusively within cleanroom.
- Small articles should be passed through double-door interlocked hatches or pass-throughs to reduce avoidable traffic.
- Install communication systems at convenient locations.
- Plant rooms and booster blowers should be as far away as possible to avoid transmission of noise and vibration.
- Ceilings should permit walking and access to overhead filters, housings and ducts.
- The design should withstand breach of the environment without detrimental effects. It must allow access for maintenance, both preventive and repair, without violation of air quality after the system has returned to normal mode.
- Prioritise and lay out work along a clean-to-dirty axis, positioning the most critical operations closest to the cleanest zone in the room.
- Base location of entry and exit points on logistic considerations such that operator movements and travel are minimised.
- Care should be taken not to exceed building structural stress limits at the site selected and reinforcement should be provided where necessary.

The manner in which the cleanroom shell is constructed and maintained, and the choice of materials that go into its making, will have a significant influence on the ultimate performance of the facility.

- All internal surfaces should be smooth and free from cracks, ledges and cavities.
- Every part of the cleanroom should not only be cleanable, but also be easily accessible to clean and disinfect
- Corners should be reduced and rounded. Sharp corners should be avoided.
- Among the important criteria for choice of materials for use in cleanroom shell construction are:
    - Flammability & fire-retardancy
    - Reactivity
    - Corrosivity
    - Toxicity
    - Low static, preferably antistatic or conductive
    - Low outgassing of adsorbed gases and vapours
    - Low particle-shedding & sloughing
    - High water repellency & ability to inhibit microbial growth
    - Cleanability
    - Ability to withstand cleaning & disinfecting agents
    - All permanent pipes and cables should be boxed in.
- All fittings should be flush. Only those which are essential to the operation being carried out are to be fitted within the room. All other fittings such as fuse boxes, switch panels, isolators and valves should be located outside.
- Furniture, production and test equipment, lighting and lifting devices should be designed, manufactured and installed in a manner such that generation of dust particles or other contaminants is kept to the bare minimum.
- Appropriately sited control pressure relief grilles or flaps should be provided in cases when it is needed to ensure that overpressure is bled to atmosphere (if necessary, through adjacent change rooms and ante-rooms).
- To avoid claustrophobia and enhance aesthetics, be generous with view panels. Do not fit on external walls. View panels should be double-glazed and sealed to minimise heat transfer, aid sound proofing and serve as back up seal in the event either pane requires replacement.

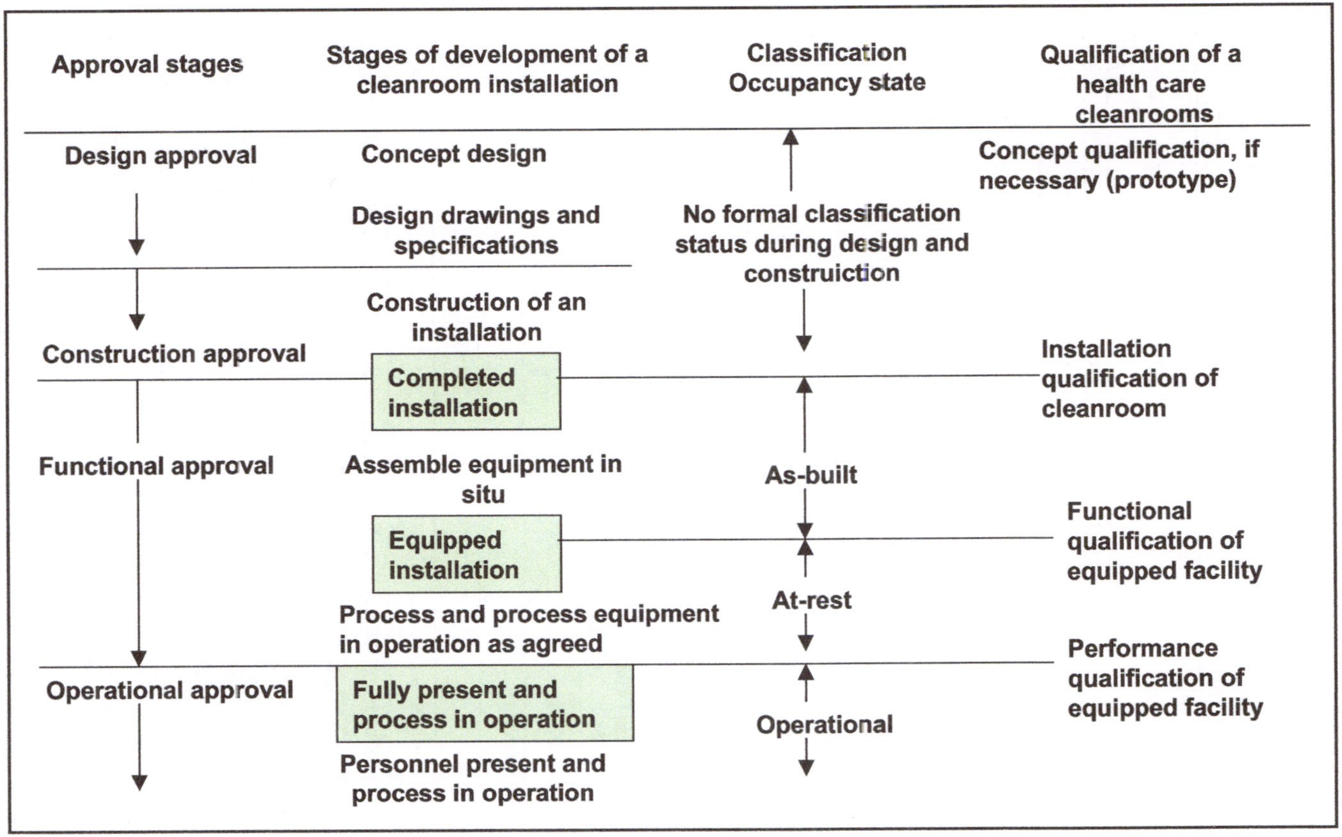

Fig. 3.26: Project flow chart as described in DIS:ISO 14644-4

Materials	Electrostatic Control	Abrasion resistance	Impact resistance	Outgassing
Walls				
Anodized aluminium	Poor	Good	No	Low
Coated metals	Poor/ fair/ good	Good	Medium to low	Low to high
Flexible curtains/walls	Poor/fair	Low	Good	Medium to high
Glass	Poor	Good	No	Low
Glass with conductive coating	Good	Good	No	Low
Plastic laminates an sheets applied to substrate	Poor/fair/good	Good	Fair	Medium to high
Resin panels, e.g. phenolic / polyester	Poor/fair/good	good	Fair	Medium to high
Stainless Steel	Good	Good	Good	Very low
Transparent polymer with conducive coating	Good	Low	Fair	Low to medium
Transparent polymers, e.g. polycarbonate, PMMA	Poor	Low	Fair	Low to medium
Ceiling(s)				
Anodized aluminium	Poor	Good	No	low
Coated metals	Poor/fair/good	Good	Medium to low	Low to high
Plasti laminates and sheets applied to substrate	Poor/fair/good	Good	Fair	Medium to high
Resin panels, e.g. phenolic / polyester	Poor/fair/good	Good	Fair	Medium to high
Stainless Steel	Good	Good	Good	Very low
Transparent polymer with conductive coating	Good	Low	Fair	Low to medium
Transparent polymers, e.g. polycarbonate, PMMA	Poor	Low	Fair	Low to medium
Floors				
Anodized aluminium (raised floor)	Poor	Good	Low	Low
Coated metals	Poor/fair/good	Good	Medium to low	Low to high
Cut polished stone/terrazzo	Poor/fair	Good	Good	Low
Glass	Poor	Good	No	Low
Glass with conductive coating	Good	Good	No	Low
Insitu epoxy coating	Poor/fair/good	Fair	Fair	Low to high
Plastic laminates and sheets applied to substrate	Poor/fair/good	Good	Fair	Medium to high
Resin panles, e.g. phenolic / polyester	Poor/fair/good	Good	Fair	Medium to high
Stainless Steel (raised floor)	Good	Good	Good	Very Low
Tiles	Poor/fair	Good	Good	Low
Transparent polymer with conductive coating	Good	Low	Fair	Low to medium
Transparent polymers, e.g. polycarbonate, PMMA	Poor	Low	Fair	Low to medium

NOTE 1 All the above mentioned materials meet basic requirements such as non-shedding and cleanability
NOTE 2 In the electrostatic column, the elements have been qualified as follows : good = conductive, fair = dissipative, poor = non-conductive.

Fig. 3.27: Characteristics of common cleanroom construction materials as described in DIS:ISO: 14644-4

The air entrapped between the panes will expand and contract; hence fit filtered *breathers* that aspirate from the cleanroom side.

- Care must be taken during planning and installation to ensure that utilities are not located in close juxtaposition to one another, so that at the time when repairs are undertaken on one, the inevitable fall out of contaminants does not compromise the integrity of the rest.
- False ceilings to reduce the effective room volume is a common feature, but when used inside clean rooms additional care must be taken not only to provide access for cleaning, but also to *make sure that they are in deed cleaned thoroughly at regular intervals*. Sporadic *showers* of contaminants from the ceiling are not uncommon, and they can nullify all the good work put in else where. False ceilings should be sealed to prevent ingress of contaminants; but remember that sealing the gaps in the ceiling tiles can be a tricky job: more easily said than done. For this reason, most designers favour a walkable ceiling which obviates the need to access the overhead portion from within the cleanroom.
- A warning system should be installed to warn of failure in the air supply.

Cleanroom Construction Protocol : Build Clean Concept

Increasingly, more attention is being paid today to the quality of starting materials, as evidenced by the greater focus on Active Process Ingredients, for example. This is in line with the general philosophy "well begun is half done". In building a clean facility, if you start clean, chances are you will be on stream a lot quicker than if you did not.

Cleanroom Construction Protocol, the basic document that governs job-site construction procedures, is designed to bring a state-of-the art cleanroom on line as quickly as possible. It represents a radical departure from standard/ normal construction techniques and practices. An integrated approach involving design, construction, planning, and erection through joint training & enforced implementation.

Training in basic cleanroom construction protocol should be provided to all participating personnel: architects, contractors, equipment & process engineers, technicians, facility managers, other managers etc

The objectives are :

- Designers must plan a facility that lends itself to clean installation
- Construction supervisors must plan the construction sequence
- Construction workers must not only learn cleanroom concepts and techniques, but also believe in their necessity

- Client must recognise that there are costs as well as benefits associated with working clean
- Material suppliers must fulfill the requirements of specifications, including those relating to packaging and shipping.
- Clean envelope boundaries are usually established after the steel structure has been painted & concrete work has been sealed
- Painstakingly maintained during construction
- Temporary construction personnel air locks and gowning areas established
- Limit to only one entry point to the clean envelope
- All materials and tools entering cleanroom envelope should be cleaned and inspected
- Ideally construction tools and equipments brought into clean envelope should remain there for the project's duration
- Structural sub-assemblies shall be cleaned in the materials lock before bringing into clean space for installation
- Air handling units should be installed and commissioned
- Thoroughly clean HVAC system
- Blow down prefiltered air
- Clean room construction begins with the training of the contractors. It is important for them to understand not only that we want it clean, but why, as a step toward both quality and education
- Build a temporary "cleanroom" to store all raw materials. These materials should be wiped using isopropyl alcohol and then sealed before taking them into clean envelope
- Once concrete is poured, workers are required to wear booties when entering the shell of the building
- During stud and duct work on the shell of the cleanroom workers are required wear cleanroom gloves
- At the time of installing equipment workers should wear full face masks, head gear, booties & bunny suits
- Traffic in the building shall be strictly controlled

- Every piece of equipment brought into the fab shall pass through material staging area where it is cleaned using IPA and then enter the main cleanroom
- The cleanroom envelope, material air lock, personnel air locks & air showers shall be established first
- Material air lock shall be large enough for removal of packing material and cleaning
- Personnel air locks shall be large enough to provide for garments and shoe storage
- A laydown area is provided for cleanroom construction materials delivered to the site
- A laydown area inside clean envelope for storing materials that have been cleaned and ready for use

Phase I : "Gross" condition of cleanliness

This includes all basic construction work involving

- Overhead fixtures like plumbing, HVAC, Chemical exhaust ducts, HEPA unit holders
- Walls
- DI water lines
- Bulk gas lines
- In house vacuum systems
- Flooring etc
- Some process equipment protected by plastic wrap

During this phase the entire area shall be vacuumed twice a day. Initial HVAC blowdowns mark the end of this phase, after which most remaining potential particle generating operations like drilling, sawing, duct fabrication and pipe assembly commences outside the clean envelope.

Phase II : Intermediate conditions of cleanliness

This period includes cleaning of all walls, plumbing components, electrical conduits, HVAC ducts, installation of HEPA filters. Plastic wraps on already installed equipment are wiped and carefully removed; equipment wiped with IPA using cleanroom wiper

Note: Proper gowning procedure shall be observed by employees involved in this cleaning operation and in the assembly of modular HEPA units

Phase III : Precision cleaning

Governing procedures during this phase shall conform to ISO 5 (Class 100) standards. Any additional equipment arriving wrapped (plastic) shall be transported to ISO 7 (Class 10,000) staging room. Procedures for unpacking, wipe down and cleaning of equipment are laid down and followed.

Molecular contaminants shed by building materials of a cleanroom result in the "sick building syndrome". Chemical aggression is introduced from every gram of material used in the construction of a cleanroom. This is due to "degassing" by synthetic and organic materials.

Sources of molecular contaminants in a cleanroom

- Brick, mortar
- Surface roughness
- HEPA ceiling system
- Process tooling
- Human beings
- Low molecular weight aerosols
- Gas phase substances through make up air

Large ionic species producers

- Copper & aluminium cooling / heating coils
- Bare metallic surfaces (GI sheet metal, steel etc,)
- Tungsten electrodes of ionisation systems
- Xylene. A product in paints & caulks
- Mass flow of ionic contaminents from makeup air
- Gel seal systems of HEPA grid and ceiling system
- Surface roughness

Guidelines for personnel working within the clean envelope should cover

- use of cleanroom garments
- personnel behaviour
- break and lunch procedures
- logistics associated with personal articles
- personal clean down
- clean tools storage

- other activities
- formal orientation programme all persons working within clean envelope must undergo

Clean envelope construction operations requiring permit

A permit must be granted only after the contractor/sub-contractor demonstrates his ability to comply with the requirements of Cleanroom Construction Protocol.

- drilling
- welding
- painting
- cutting
- grinding
- soldering
- filing
- Other "dirty" operations

Cleanroom Construction Protocol has been widely adopted in semicon fabrication facilities that aspire for environment classification of ISO 5 and better; but most others, specially those setting up less stringent environments, regard it as a wholly impractical and expensive concept. The protocol has been mentioned here for you to adopt, adapt or modify to suit your requirements.

4 Air Filters

In environmental control design there comes a point where some means of contaminant removal from a stream of air is required. Filtration is an important building block on which the concept of environment control is built. An understanding of filtration principles, filter grades and capacities, and methods of comparing performance is desirable to assist in the consideration of facility selection and design for specific purposes.

Air filters are devices that help remove matter suspended in air. They vary in size, shape, capacity and the method by which they function. In this section we look at various types in use, consider their relative strengths and weaknesses and lay down the foundation for intelligent selection, use and qualification.

Few disciplines compare with the profusion of nomenclature that abounds in air filtration technology. Names are given on the basis of how they work; how they are made; the filtering medium; the intended application; the location where fitted; acronyms and brands.

In an *electrostatic air filter*, air is passed through a strong electrostatic field, which imparts a charge to the suspended contaminants. The charged particles are then deposited on collector plates carrying the opposite charge.

Table 4.1

How does it work? (Type)	With what is it made? (Medium)	How is it made? (Execution)	What is its purpose? (Application)
Mechanical Electrostatic Electronic Chemical	Microfibreglass Glass wool Sintered glass Charcoal Dry fabric Oil wetted fabric PU foam Membrane Silica Lithium chloride	Flange Cassette Box Sandwich Disk Pleated Minipleat Separatorless Gradvel	Prefilter Coarse filter Final filter Fine filter Intermediate filter
Where is it fitted? (Location)	**Descriptive** (Function/ Acronym)	**Brand** (Make)	**Grade** (Test)
Bank Terminal Ceiling Fresh air Exhaust	Depth Fire-retardant Fire-resistant VLSI HEPA ULPA	Flanders Cambridge Vokes Microvee Absolute Ultraklenz	Type A Type B Type C Type D Grade I Grade II

Efficiency declines with use. It is relatively effective in removal of smaller particles, but less efficient with larger; contaminants break loose from the collector plates and re-entrain in the air stream causing sudden spikes of contamination; the system chatters; requires frequent cleaning and maintenance; causes arcing, corona discharge and releases ozone. Usage is generally restricted to Class M6.5 (100,000) environments like telephone exchanges.

Radiation from naturally occurring radioactive materials in the earth's crust and in the air and cosmic radiation strip electrons from molecules in the air leaving positive ions behind. Positive ions are formed at the rate of about 10 per cc per sec. Recombination does not proceed at a very rapid rate because the returning electron often misses the parent molecule, and may ultimately attach itself to some other molecule thereby creating a negative ion. Thus the ion concentration increases with time until an equilibrium level is reached. An atmospheric ion concentration of 2700 ions per cc would be considered a

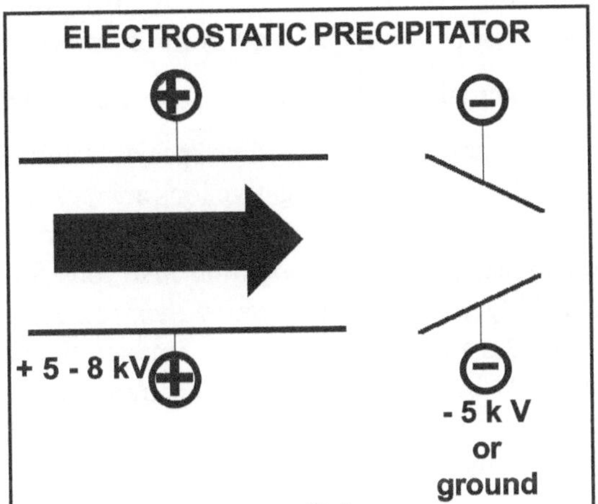

1. Lower start-up efficiency as compared to HEPA
2. High efficiency at sub-micronic levels, relatively ineffective with larger particles
3. Arcing releases ozone
4. Requires frequent cleaning to maintain efficiency
5. Charged particles escaping can cause damage downstream
6. Arcing causes temporary localised loss of efficiency, resulting in release of collected contaminants

Fig. 4.1

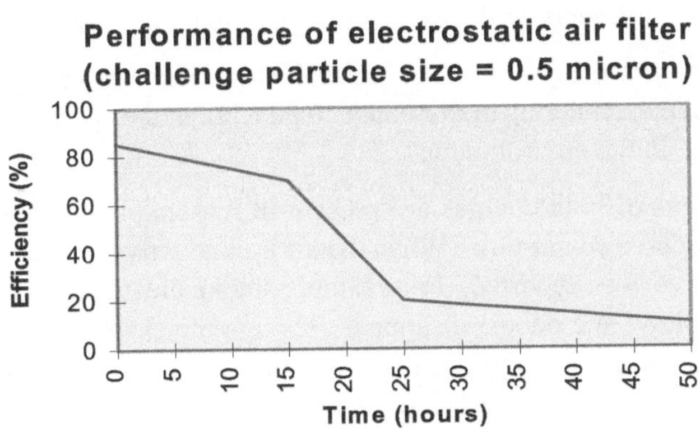

Fig. 4.2

high natural level. In practice the concentration varies between 1000 to 2000 ions per cc, or about one ion for every 10^{13} molecules.

Instruments are available with Limits of Detection down to 20 ions per cc.

Oxygen molecules apparently have some special affinity for stray electrons, and as a result nearly all observed negative ions are oxygen molecules with an extra electron. In contrast, positive ions are found in almost all gases, though carbon dioxide appears to be most common. All ions form clumps of other molecules, especially water vapour, around themselves. Positive ions form the larger clumps. As a result of their being smaller, the negative ion clumps have greater mobility. In dry air, the negative ion moves at speeds approximately 1.2 times that of a positive ion; but as humidity increases, the speeds diminish and approach each other.

Ionic imbalance in the air results in static charges, which cannot only prove a fire hazard but also damage sensitive CMOS circuits. Many believe that an excess of negative ions is beneficial, but from the process view point, either charge in excess is equally unacceptable.

The mobility of the ion has a direct bearing on the influence it wields in contamination control, as a potential contaminant itself, or in assisting in the control process by aiding static charge removal.

Static charges should always be discharged through controlled resistance, direct shorting can produce large currents that zap components. Many of us who have touched metallic doorknobs in cold dry conditions have experienced the jolt caused by such discharge. Unless controlled, charged molecules tend to yield up their charge to walls, floors, ceilings and any object they encounter. Their motion in air may be caused by electrostatic forces of attraction or repulsion; bombardments or diffusion through a boundary layer.

Electronic air filters or bi-phasic sequential multinodal ionisers, quite unlike electrostatic filters, rendering the air conductive, without the altering the overall charge balance in the environment.

Wherever ions of both charges are present in reasonably close proximity, the zone is rendered *conductive*. When the air is conductive, some interesting phenomena have been reported. For example smoke clears out; bacteria and viruses die rapidly; and odours disappear. Though the exact modus operandi is still unclear, one theory suggests that when the oxygen molecule accepts an extra electron its chemical behaviour changes, rendering it more aggressive than normal. The products of incomplete combustion that constitute smoke are fully oxidised; cell proteins and enzymes are denatured; and aromatic rings

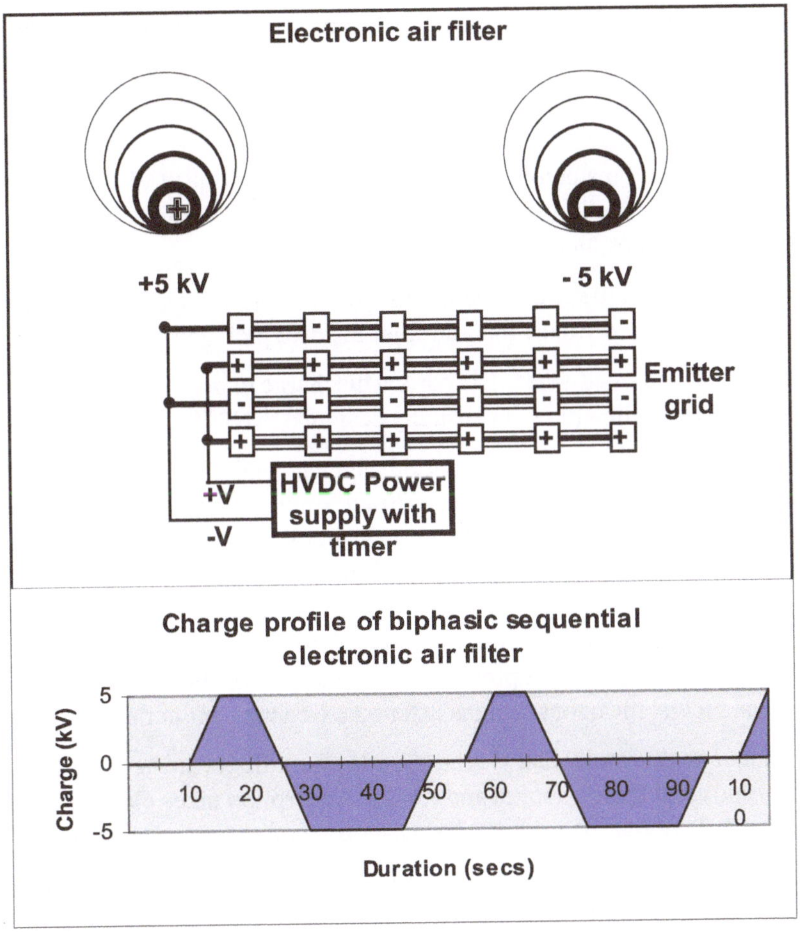

Fig. 4.3

are broken down to aliphatic chains. If there are any charged contaminants in this zone, they will gravitate toward the node that attracts and tamely (and harmlessly) yield up their charge.

The simplest electronic filtration system utilises high voltage AC fed to sharp needlelike emitters; the next stage of refinement uses HVDC.

Bi-phasic sequential pulsing with relaxation or recovery intervals is more advanced; using sensors for monitoring the ambient ionic balance in a feedback loop is state-of-the-art. Electronic filters are used almost exclusively for static charge control, though as mentioned earlier, they also help in significantly reducing ambient bioburden, odour and vapour levels.

Cleanroom Air Ionisers: The generation and storage of electrostatic charge in an Electronic Processing Area (EPA) occurs primarily on insulators and isolated conductors. Many conductors can be grounded by conventional techniques, but insulators cannot.

Where possible, insulators should be eliminated from the EPA but where this is impossible the ions emitted by an ioniser can eliminate both negative and positive charges on an insulator.

Ionisers may also be used where conventional grounding of conductors is impractical or very difficult for example, inside a pick and place machine.

Ionisers feature steady-state DC corona discharge to provide high ion output and low recombination rates, and usually designed to NIST traceable standards.

All ioniser emitter points require periodic maintenance. The small electrostatic field that creates air ionisation can attract small particles or interact with chemicals in the air. If deposits form on the emitter points, they are usually removed by wiping with a swab or cloth moistened with isopropyl alcohol (IPA) or methanol. The maintenance interval depends on the characteristics of the cleanroom or production area, and each ionisation user must determine the appropriate maintenance programme. Some ionisers however are easier to clean than others: the better designs offer quick-change emitter point cassettes.

Chemical filters, molecular sieves and adsorbent filters are used for removal of hazardous and toxic vapours and fumes. Adsorption takes place at external surfaces; diffusion at phase boundaries - intracrystalline and pore diffusion.

Filtration efficiency is almost 100% up to the filter's *escape* threshold, after which it declines rapidly to near zero. Chemical filters can trap contaminants at concentrations as low as 10 ppm up to slugs of 10,000 ppm. Higher the boiling point of the contaminant, the greater is the weight that is absorbed. Generally they are more effective in removal of organic, and less so with inorganic substances. 1 gm of a typical chemical filter like activated carbon made from coconut shell has a surface area available for adsorption of 800-1100 sq metres.

Fibrous filters: Particle filters for contamination control applications in manufacturing environments are predominantly of the *fibrous* type. Other types of air filters have not been widely applied due either to lower efficiency, higher initial cost, problems of maintenance, or the narrow size ranges in which they are really effective. Fibrous filters, also commonly called *mechanical* filters, trap suspended contaminants by bringing to play several different mechanisms.

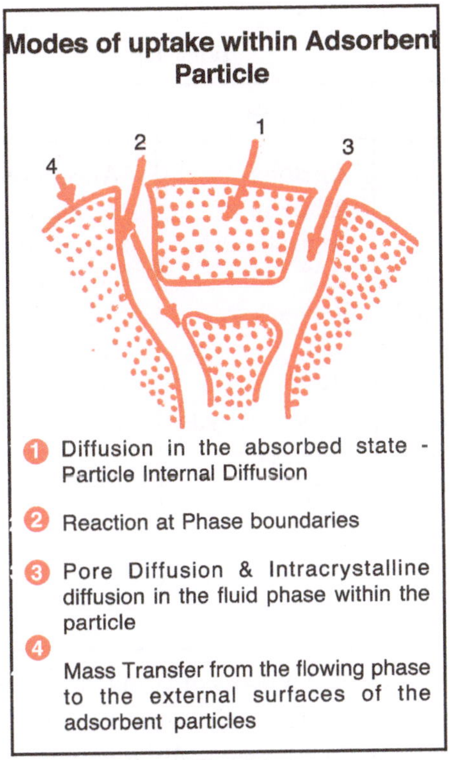
Modes of uptake within Adsorbent Particle
1
2
3
4
1 Diffusion in the absorbed state - Particle Internal Diffusion
2 Reaction at Phase boundaries
3 Pore Diffusion & Intracrystalline diffusion in the fluid phase within the particle
4 Mass Transfer from the flowing phase to the external surfaces of the adsorbent particles

Fig. 4.4

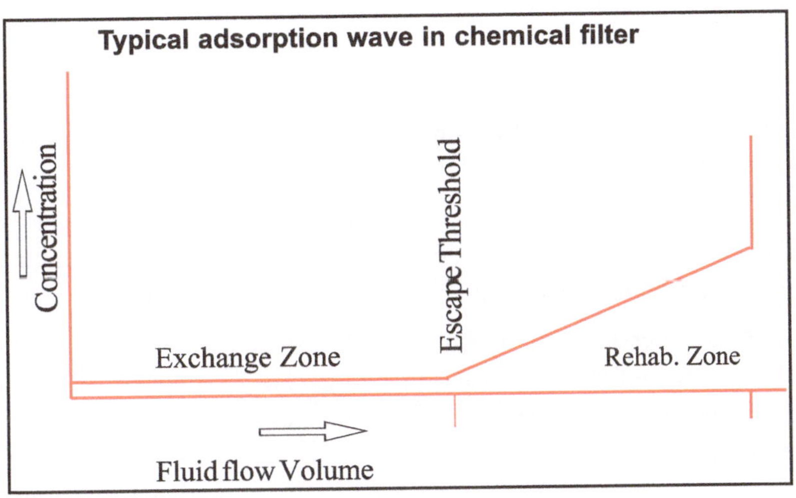
Typical adsorption wave in chemical filter
Concentration
Escape Threshold
Exchange Zone
Rehab. Zone
Fluid flow Volume

Fig. 4.5

Table 4.2

High	Medium	Fair	Low
Acetic Acid	Acetone	Acetaldehyde	CO
Alcohol	Aerolein	Amines	CO_2
Benzene	Anaesthetics	Ammonia	NO
Odours	H_2S	Formaldehyde	H_2
Butyl Alcohol	Solvents	HCl	C_2H_2
Caprylic Acid	Cl_2	HF	CH_4
CCL_4	HCN	SO_2	
Chloropicrin	Butyraldehyde	NO_2	
Mercaptans	Phosgene		
Ethyl Acetate	SO_3		
Pheno	Pyridine		
Toluene			
Turpentine			

Sifting is the first of them, a process of go-no go where larger particles are prevented from passing through the air pathways of the filter. The larger the size of the particle, the more efficient is filtration through sifting.

Sedimentation, the balance between gravitational forces and viscous drag of air, causes particles to settle out. Again, the larger the particle, the higher the sedimentation rate.

Inertial forces play an important part when the air is constrained to follow convoluted paths. The longer the path and greater the sharp bends, the higher is the efficiency of filtration through inertial effects.

Impaction is the head-on collision of a particle on the filter media at a spot where there is no air pathway. Such impingement reduces the particle kinetic energy of motion to zero, leaving it stranded at the point of impact.

A Fibre filter surface, specially on the upstream side, is covered with tiny follicles that tend to trip a particle in motion. This is *interception*. In addition, the aerodynamic pressures cause these follicles to fibrillate, thus augmenting interception efficiency.

Coalescence is coming together of tiny particles charged oppositely; *agglomeration* is the same process, but featuring neutral particles that bind through physical attraction caused by cohesive or adhesive forces. As a net result the particles grow large enough to be trapped by other mechanisms.

Diffusion is caused by Brownian effects causing tiny particles to move randomly away from air stream flow direction, causing it to leave the stream altogether and be trapped.

Electrostatic charges cause charged particles to deviate from and often leave the flow stream.

Surface tension effects produce *capillary action* to draw small particles away from the air stream.

Surface adsorption often helps remove contaminants in the gaseous or vapour phases.

In addition to efficiency, the relative performance of a filter is influenced by its ability to retain particles that are trapped and its dust holding capacity. The sloughing off of particles is a question of reliability which must be weighed in while economically evaluating a filter. Likewise, rapid clogging of a filter, even though highly efficient, would be unprofitable. The mechanism that affects filter sloughing and clogging are the aerosol velocity at the filter fibres, the particle size distribution and concentration of the aerosol, the physical phase of the aerosol, and the characteristics of the filter media. The filter characteristics affecting retention and clogging performance are the type of fibre (monofilament vs high nap), the fibre diameter (greater surface area for deposition for a given filter porosity), the assembly of the fibres (a coherent cloth filter clogs more rapidly than a flocculent felt material), the porosity of the fibre assembly, and the depth of the filter media.

There are two generic classes of fibrous filters - viscous impingement type and the dry type, which are commonly used in factory environments. Both are *true* filters in that the pressure drop increases with dust loading to an operating point at which they are cleaned sufficiently for reuse, or replaced.

Impingement filters are generally constructed of coarse fibres arranged in a porous bed to operate at high velocities (250-700 fpm) through the media at a low pressure drop. Filter face velocities of 300-500 fpm are common. Particle deposition and retention is aided by the application of a viscous substance to the media. The media may be glass, hair, synthetic fibre, plastic foams, or metal mesh. Such filters are often used as prefilters in a multi-filter system, being of low cost, low pressure drop, and more effective in the capture and retention of larger particles and lint.

Table 4.3: Comparison of Cleanroom and HVAC filters

	Cleanroom Filters	HVAC Filters
Efficiency	99.99 – 99.99999+%	65 – 99.97%
Flow Rates	<100CFM/SqFt	> 200 cfm/sq ft
Media Velocity	1 – 5 fpm	5 – 12 fpm
Size	24 x 48 in	24 x 24
Life	Upto 10+ years	1 year or less
Location	Final air delivery	Central air

Table 4.4 Correlation between classifications based on fractional efficiency of fine and coarse filters - Euro and American Standards

EUROVENT 4/9 CLASS	AVERAGE % Arrestance using Synthetic Dust	ANSI/ASHRAE 52.1 % Efficiency 0.4 mm particles	CEN* EN779 Class	EVALUATION METHODS Tests @ I m³ / sec
EU 1	$A_m < 65$		G 1	Gravimetric
EU 2	$65 < A_m < 80$		G 2	250 Pa Final Loss
EU 3	$80 < A_m < 90$		G 3	
EU 4	$90 < A_m$		G 4	
EU 5		$40 < E_m < 60$	F 5	Opacimetric
EU 6		$60 < E_m < 80$	F 6	450 Pa Final Loss
EU 7		$80 < E_m < 90$	F 7	
EU 8		$90 < E_m < 95$	F 8	
EU 9		$95 < E_m$	F 9	

* *Comitte Europeen du Normalisation*

Table 4.5: Eurovent Classification of High Efficiency air filters

Class	Filter Efficiency (E_i%)
EU10	$95<E_i<99.9$
EU11	$99.9<E_i<99.97$
EU12	$99.97<E_i<99.99$
EU13	$99.99<E_i<99.999$
EU14	$99.999<E_i$

Table 4.6 : Co-relation based on Deutsche Industrie Normen Schwebstoff - HEPA and ULPA - range and American National Standards

EUROVENT 4/4	TG/195 EN 1822 & DIN 24183	INITIAL EFFICIENCY Ei % IES-RP	PENETRATION % IES-RP	INTEGRAL EFFICIENCY % at MPPS
EU 10	H 10	95 < Ei < 99.9	5 > P > 0.1	85
EU 11	H 11	99.9 < Ei < 99.97	0.1 > P > 0.03	95
EU 12	H 12	99.97<Ei < 99.99	0.03 > P > 0.01	99.5
EU 13	H 13	99.99<Ei<99.999	0.01 > P > 0.001	99.95
EU 14	H 14	99.999 < Ei	0.001 > P	99.995
EU 15	U 15	99.9975		99.9995
EU 16	U 16	99.99975		99.99995
EU 17	U 17	99.999975		99.999995

Table 4.7: Eurovent Ratings of High Efficiency air filters

CEN Class	Efficiency MPPS (%)	Leak test local (%)	Penetration Ratio	Leak test method
H10	85	-	-	visible
H11	95	-	-	visible/scanning MPPS
H12	99.5	97.5	> 5	visible/scanning MPPS
H13	99.95	99.75	> 5	scanning MPPS
H14	99.995	99.975	> 5	scanning MPPS
U15	99.9995	99.9975	> 5	scanning MPPS
U16	99.99995	99.99975	> 5	scanning MPPS
U17	99.999995	99.9999	> 20	scanning MPPS

Dry type filters differ from viscous impingement type in the use of smaller diameter fibres which are more densely spaced in the blanket media. Also, the viscous coating is not applied to the fibres. The media mats or paper-like blankets may be composed of fine glass fibres, cellulose, wool felts, asbestos, or synthetic fibres. The filament diameters range from 10 microns to sub-micronic dimensions. Approach velocities to the filter of 250-625 fpm are commonly used, but the velocity through the media range from 2-90 fpm. The low media filtration velocities allow diffusion effects to be pronounced. The closely interwoven small diameter fibres create the convolutions in the air pathway. Thus dry type filter construction is commonly used for intermediate and high efficiency systems where the capture of small particles is sufficiently important to compensate for their higher cost, lower dust holding capacity and higher operating pressure losses. The highest quality dry type design - the HEPA and ULPA filters - are constructed to be fail-safe as far as sloughing is concerned.

HEPA & ULPA filters

High Efficiency Particulate Arrestors, or HEPA filters, were developed under a classified US Government contract by Arthur D Little, a Cambridge, Massachusetts research and development company in the early 1940s. Until that time, high efficiency filtration was achieved by filling the air ducts in the laboratory with glass fibrous packing material. This system required inordinate amounts of packing material in long sections of duct, causing pressure drops so high that compressors were required to move the air. With the declassification of the technology came improvements in efficiency, performance and safety. The development of new filtration media was slow until 1975, but progressed at a dramatic pace thereafter with the rapid expansion in demand for higher and higher performance requirements.

Filtration media for use in rigid frame dry type filtration devices are generally categorised into four groups which describe filtration efficiency: standard prefilters, super prefilters, HEPAs and ULPAs. Design of filtration efficiency is generally accomplished by the selection of appropriate glass microfibres, the mean diameter of which ranges from 0.26 to 7.0 microns. These filtration products consist of 100% glass fibre containing approximately 5% (by weight) acrylic binder. The binder is necessary to give the media sufficient strength to be easily pleated on a wide variety of equipment and still have sufficient integrity to be fabricated into a filter element. All filtration media of this type are closely controlled blends of several blends of several glass fibres. A HEPA grade media would have a much higher percentage of fine diameter fibres, and an ULPA grade an even higher one, than prefilters, By closely controlling the percentages in each grade's formulation, the media manufacturer assures the same filtration efficiency and physical properties from roll to roll, and from batch to batch.

The filter media manufacturing process is similar to other fibre-based, non-woven, paper-like products. The raw materials (glass fibres, water, binders, chemicals) are put into a large pulper, similar to a huge mixer, where they are blended at high velocity. The resulting slurry is pumped to one of several large chests where homogeneity is maintained by continuous recirculation. Then the slurry goes to the headbox of the paper machine where it is deposited on a fine mesh, endlessly revolving screen. Water is forced through the screen by both gravity and vacuum. When the web leaves the screen, the newly formed media contains 60% to 80% water, and must be passed through a controlled drying line. As the finished product approaches the dry end of the production line it is scanned by a Betaray gauge to determine product mass, and the information is automatically fed back to a controller at the forming or wet end of the machine to compensate for any variations. The media is tested on-line to ensure that it exhibits not only sufficient physical strengths to be processed in the filter manufacturer's pleating and fabrication process, but also have the requisite filtration characteristics for its end use application.

While HEPA medium comprises very fine glass fibre filaments formed into a thin pad held in place by resin bonding agents with interstices varying in diameter from 1 to 10 microns, ULPA medium additionally features a chemically formed pad of expanded PTFE for smaller interstitial spacing. The complete specifications for HEPAs and ULPAs was given in IES-RP-CC-001 of 1986, though not carried forward with as much detail in the current version IES-RP-CC-001.3.

HEPA and ULPA filters are the basic filter elements in the design of a clean environment. The filter consists of the filter media folded into deep pleats, separated by corrugated aluminium, PVC, or any other suitable medium, and packed into a rigid frame made of treated plywood, particle board, or metal, choice being based on a balance of cost, efficiency, life, stability, and fire resistance considerations. The filter pack is cemented into the rigid frame using epoxy, PVC, rubber based or foamed sealants.

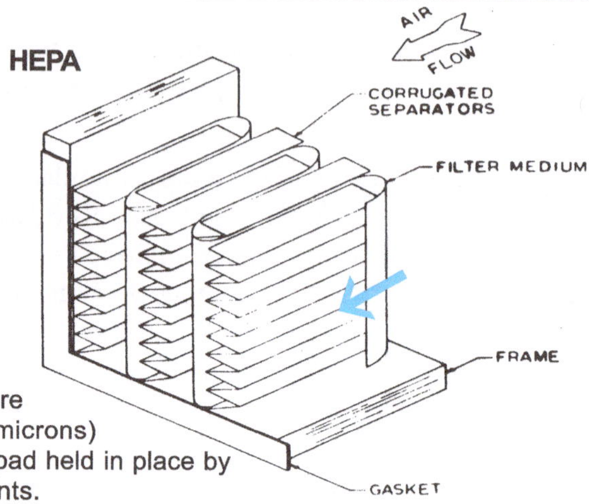

HIGH
EFFICIENCY
PARTICULATE
AIR
FILTER

HEPA MEDIUM

Very fine Glass Fibre Filaments (1-100 microns) formed into a thin pad held in place by resin bonding agents.

Interstices ... 1 - 10 microns

HEPA FILTER CONSTRUCTION

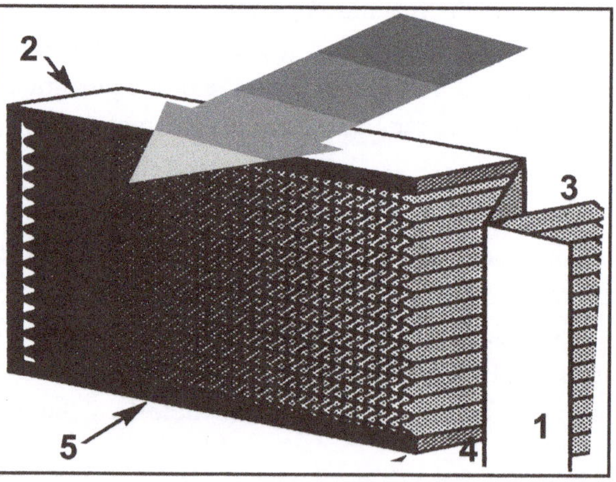

1. Glass fibre impregnated media, pleated for greater surface area
2. Frame/housing made from EGSS, anodised aluminium, painted CRCA or plywood
3. Corrugated separators of aluminium foil, mica, or PVC
4. Bonding resins - polyester, PVC, epoxy
5. Gasket - closed cell or expanded neoprene rubber

Fig.4.6

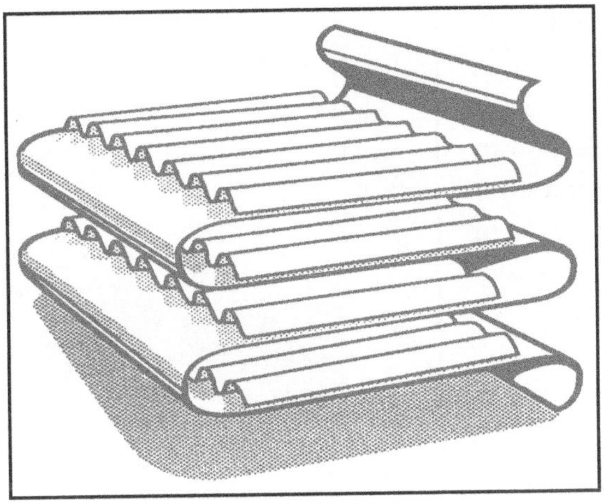

Fig. 4.7

Table 4.8

Typical media data for HEPAs and ULPAs		
Typical properties	**HEPAs**	**ULPAs**
DOP penetration, 0.3 micron @ 32 LPM/100 sq cm	0.015%	0.0001%
Pressure drop @ 32 LPM/100 sq cm	37 mm	63 mm
Basis weight	73 g/sq M	73 g/ sq M
Caliper	0.38 mm	0.38 mm
Tensile, MD	1.04 KN/M	1.04 KN/M
Tensile, CD	0.69 KN/M	0.69 KN/M
Water repellency	508 mm d'eau	508 mm d'eau
Combustible binder	5.0%	5.0%
Yield	13.7 sq M/Kg (148 sq ft/Kg)	13.7 sq M/Kg (148/sq ft/Kg)

Energy is spent in overcoming the resistance to flow offered by filters. In fluid dynamics, this is referred to as loss of pressure energy or pressure drop. The longer the air pathway, the greater is the pressure drop in mechanical and chemical filters. Electrostatic and electronic filters offer very little, if any, resistance to airflow.

Resistance to air flow through a fibrous filter is similar to air flow through a porous structure and follows D'Arcy's law. That is, the resistance to air flow varies linearly with velocity. Although as shown in Fig ., the linear relationship breaks down at higher flow rates, air flow velocities in cleanroom filter is usually well within the linear regime.

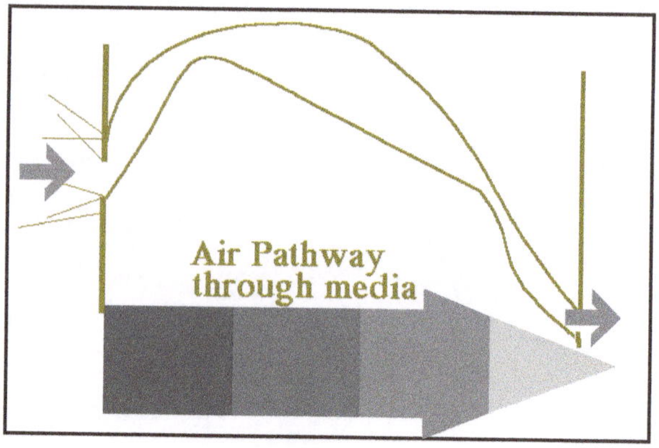

Fig. 4.8

The rated pressure drop for HEPAs is 25 mm of water column (wc) at rated airflow, although by design they should be capable of withstanding a pressure drop of 254 mm wc for 60 minutes. Normal airflow in use is generally maintained lower than rated as part of engineering over-design. Hence, at the time of installation the pressure drop across HEPAs is in the range 15 mm - 20 mm wc.

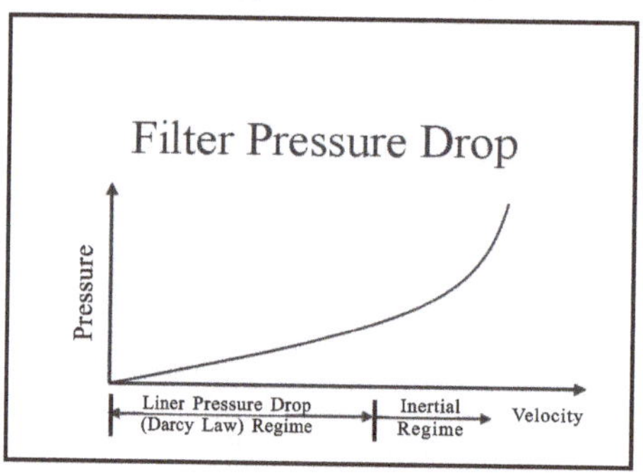

Fig. 4.9

As dirt builds up on the incident face, more resistance is offered to airflow. In other words, the pressure drop across the filter increases for the same airflow. A filter is usually deemed to have reached the end of its useful life when the pressure drop doubles in value from that at installation. An interesting observation here is that increase in filter resistance with dirt buildup implies a longer air pathway: the accumulated deposits on the incident face act as additional filters. Since efficiency improves with the length of the air pathway, *filtration actually improves with use!* A HEPA/ULPA operates at its lowest efficiency when first installed.

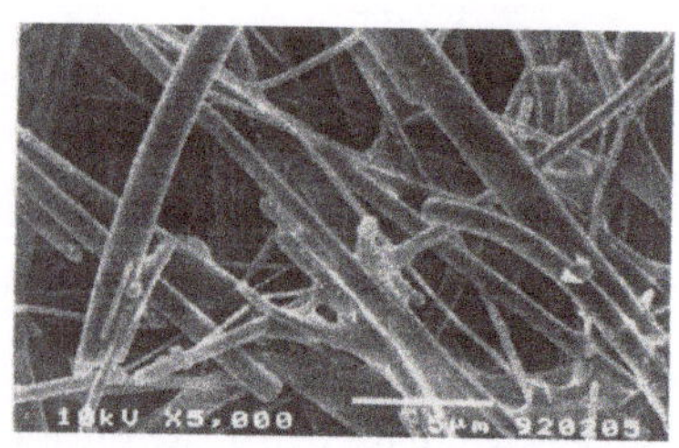

Fig. 4.10

Increasing depth of the media must not be confused with increase in pleat depth of a

Table 4.9

Filter pressure drop considerations	
Pressure drop *increases* **with**	**Pressure drop** *decreases* **with**
1. MEDIA DEPTH 2. DIRT BUILDUP 3. AIRFLOW	1. PLEAT DEPTH 2. MEDIA AREA 3. GASKET LEAK 4. MEDIA RUPTURE

pleated filter. The former increases the air pathway length, improving the probability for entrapment; whereas the latter increases the available surface of media for filtration, without affecting the media depth or air path length.

By the same token, if we increase the residence time of air in the media, chances of particle capture improves. One way to increase residence time is to reduce air velocity, or air flow. This is explained in the paragraphs that follow.

Typically, a HEPA filter of size 24" x 24" x 12" will feature media with 400 sq ft of surface area which reduces the rated approach velocity of 272 fpm down to 5 - 10 fpm (2.5 to 5 cm/sec) through the media. Note that at end of life the downstream face of the media is not stained, giving subjective proof of the filter's fail-safe nature. The velocity of air flow through the media is the most critical design parameter that affects the performance of filters. Cleanroom filters typically operate at face velocities between 75 and 100 fpm. Thus, a typical 48" x 24" cleanroom filter is designed to handle about 800 cfm, which is about half the operating velocities for HVAC filters. As shown earlier, reducing the velocity of air flow reduces the resistance linearly. However, the penetration through the media changes almost exponentially with velocity as shown in Figure 4.11. A typical ULPA media that is 99.999% efficient at 8 ft/min for 0.15 μm particles is nearly 99.99999% efficient at 2.5 ft/min.

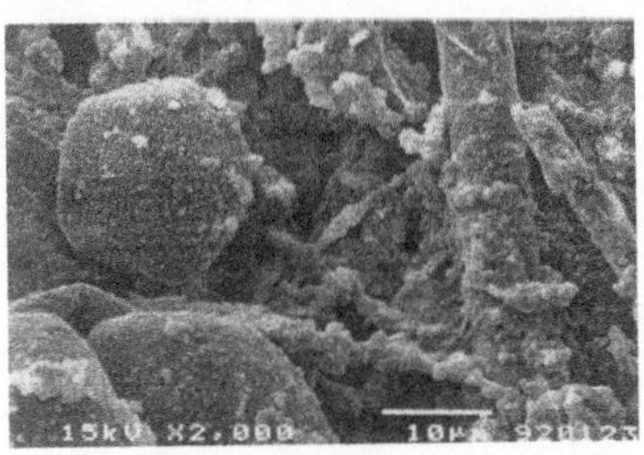

Fig. 4.11

The efficiency statement of HEPAs and ULPAs is worthy of careful interpretation. For example, a typical HEPA is claimed to remove particulates, 0.3 micron or larger, with an efficiency of 99.97%. This implies that a HEPA is not a sieve: it is not a Go - No Go device, otherwise all particles below 0.3 micron should pass (0% efficiency) and all particles 0.3 micron or larger should be arrested (100% efficiency).

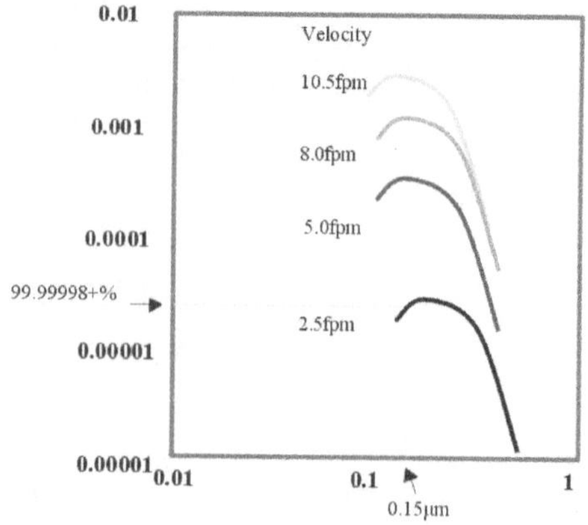

Fig. 4.12

The statement further implies that if the upstream concentration were 10,000 the downstream would show up not more than 3 particles of size 0.3 micron or larger. By extension, if the upstream count goes up to 1 million, we should find as many as 300 downstream. In other words, if the background contamination density is beyond 333,333 per cubic foot of particles 0.3 micron or larger, the downstream air cleanliness will exceed 100. *Not through any fault of the filter!*

A HEPA or ULPA is just an element offering a "controlled leak"! To understand how some larger particles escape, while some smaller particles get arrested, we re-examine the various processes at play.

The efficiency of the filter is the algebraic sum of the individual process efficiencies. The minima occurs for a HEPA in the neighbourhood of 0.3 μ, and for an ULPA in the neighbourhood of 0.12 μ . In fact the size of particles that successfully penetrate in the largest number lies in this range, where almost all processes are least efficient at capture. This range is therefore commonly referred to as the uncertainty envelope or the MPPS (maximum penetrating particles' size) regime.

If we were to cascade several HEPAs in tandem, the weakness in the MPPS regime is only further emphasised, and we are left with air enriched with particles in this size range.

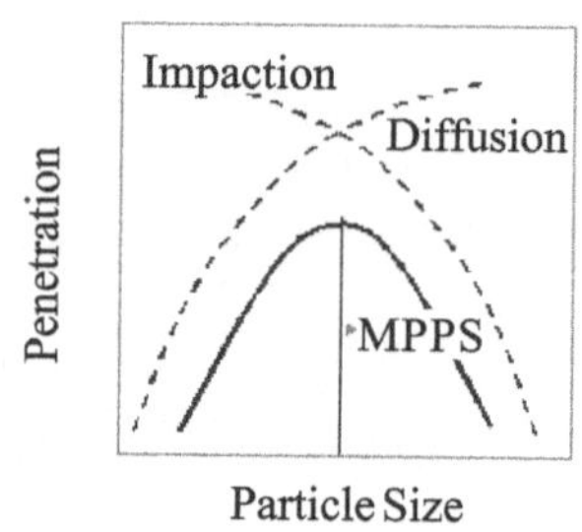

Fig. 4.13

Filters are designed for the lowest media velocity practical. Lowering velocities result in the double benefits of reduced resistance as well as increased efficiency. Reducing the

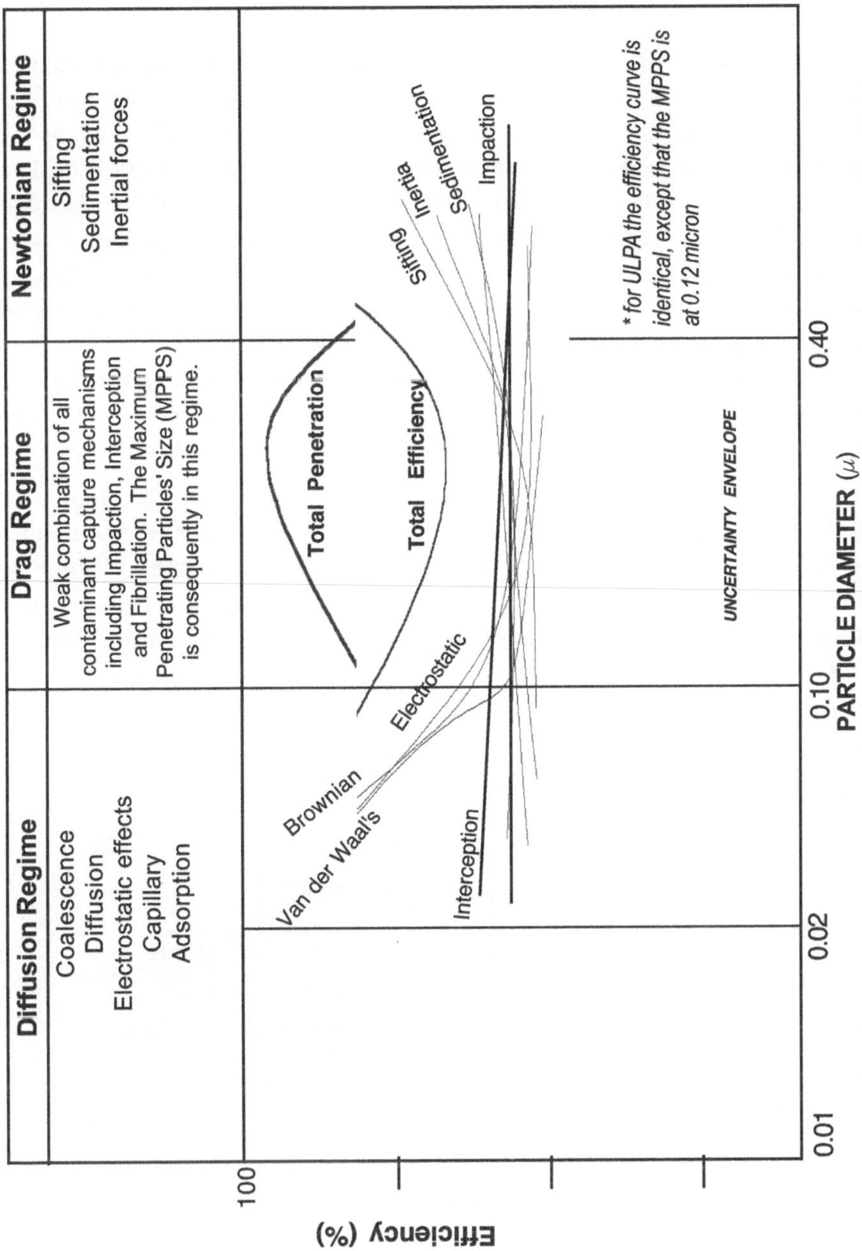

Figure 4.14 : How Particles Larger than 0.3μ Penetrate a HEPA*

velocity by half not only reduces the resistance, and consequently the energy consumption by half, it also improves the efficiency by about an order of magnitude.

The media is pleated, so that more of its surface area can be accommodated in a smaller cross-section. By increasing the surface area, we are in effect increasing the number of air pathways, so that more air can flow across the same cross-section, given the same kinetic energy. The greater the pleat depth, the greater is the surface area. The number of pleats should be specified and subsequently verified, since this is one area where competing vendors can and often do fudge. IES-RP-CC-001 of 1986 had clearly laid down the *minimum air velocity* through the filtration medium: 5 fpm. The *minimum required surface area* can then be determined by dividing the rated airflow capacity (cfm) of the filter by 5 fpm. Given the size of the rigid frame and the depth of each pleat, the number of pleats can be calculated. This aspect, too, is not as clearly spelt out in the current version IES-RP-CC-001.

The velocity through the media is adjusted by changing the amount of media contained in the filter. The amount of media in a filter is varied either by varying the pleat density (i.e., number of pleats per inch) or by varying the height of the pleated media. The pleat height is dependent more on the physical properties of the media, such as stiffness, as well as the manufacturing process. Technology is currently available to manufacture pleats as high as 12 inches.

Increasing the pleat or fold density will directly increase the media in a filter and should decrease the velocity of air flow. However, there is a limit to

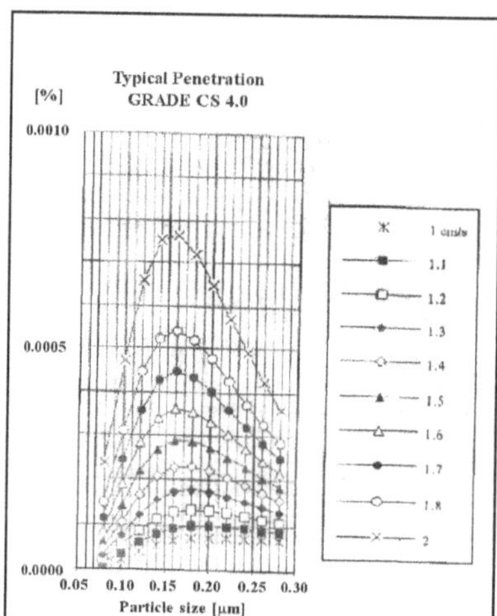

Fig. 4.15

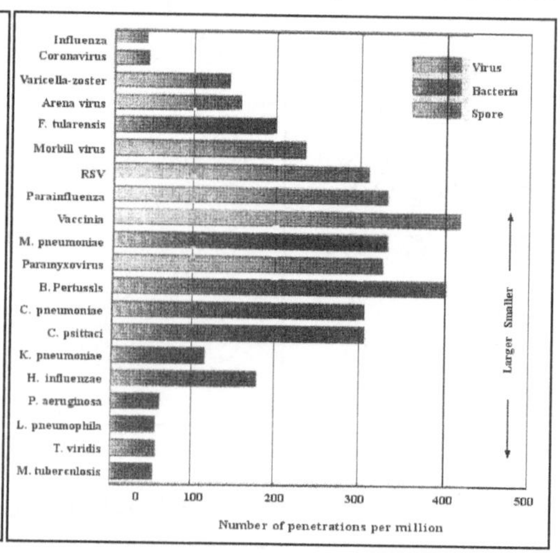

Fig. 4.16

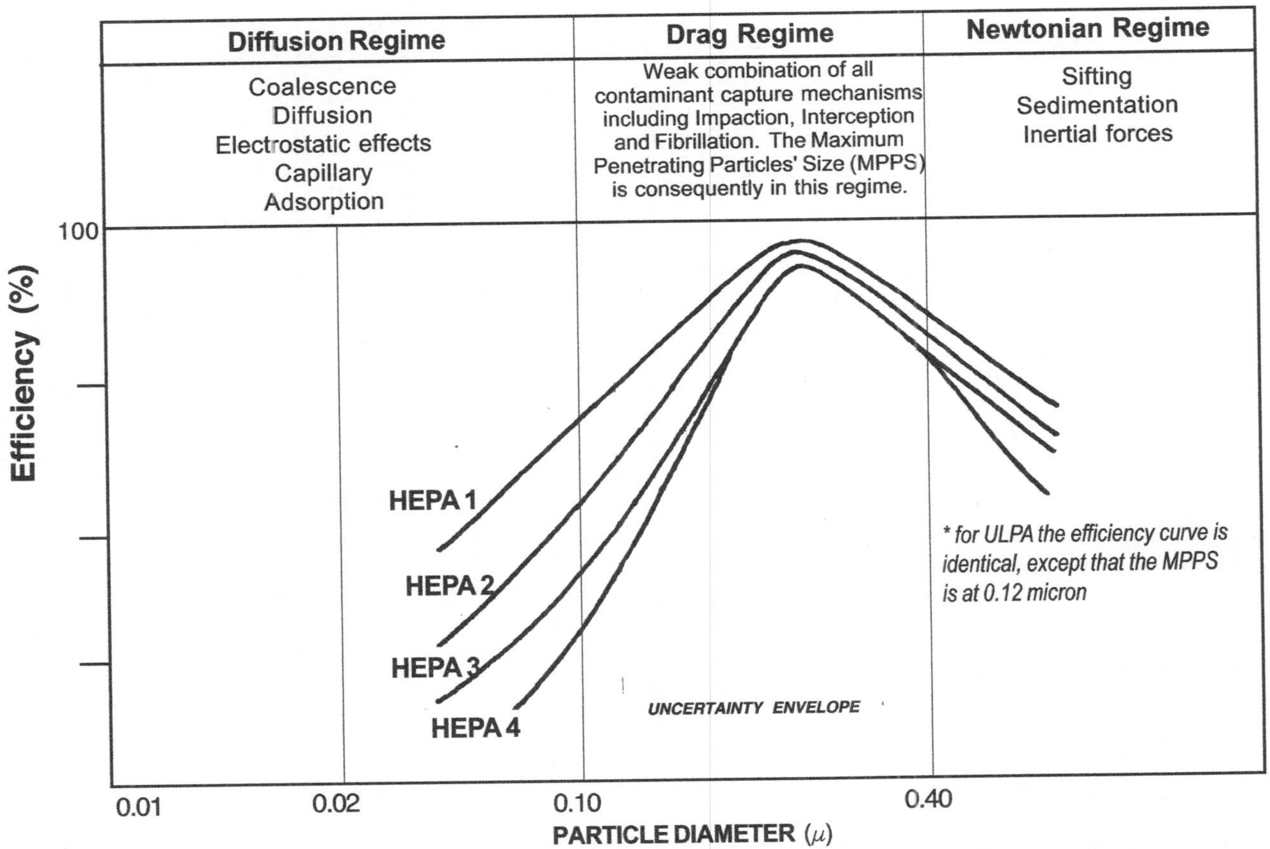

Figure 4.17 : Enrichment of MPPS and ultrafines through a cascade of HEPAs *

how close adjacent folds can be formed before the interference to flow from adjacent pleats negates any gain from increasing area of media in a filter. There is an optimum pleat density at which the resistance is the lowest. This is shown qualitatively in Figure 4.18. At lower densities there is insufficient media and at higher densities there is excess interference between adjacent pleats, causing pleat "blinding". The optimum is dependent on the media, the pleat height and filter construction.

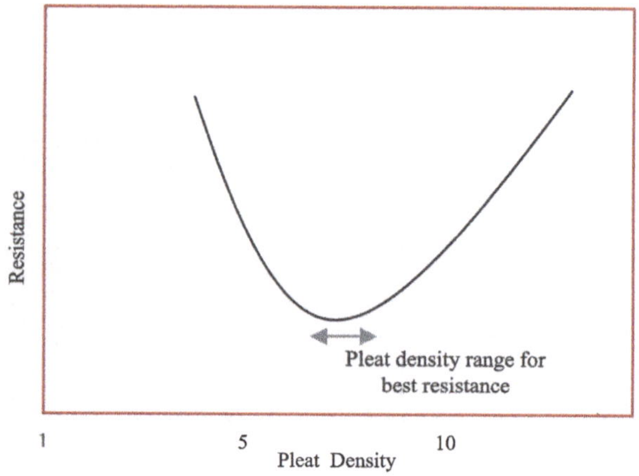

Fig. 4.18

Corrugated separators, because the media was relatively fragile. However, the presence of these separators has been a source of concern to Users of ultraclean environments because they block 20% of airflow path; abrade media; disseminate anodic particles condensates and coalesced contaminants; and cause the media to “sag” leading to bond dislodgment with age. With the introduction of stronger media with superior airflow and filtration characteristics the current trend is towards separatorless filters. Since the pleat depth is smaller with this media, filters made from it are commonly referred to as *minipleats*. In mini pleat filters, the pleats are separated either by adhesive beads, strings, or ribbons of paper applied on the media, or embossed corrugations in the media itself. Mini pleat construction allows for a greater pleat density resulting in a more compact filter than possible with separator construction for the same performance. However, due to the higher pleat density and the absence of corrugated separators to act as flow straighteners, mini pleat filters exhibit poor flow uniformity. In practice, flow uniformity is often improved by adding flow straighteners such as a face screen or media down stream of the filter.

Proper filter design requires attention to design parameters such as airflow rates, resistance, penetration, critical particle size, airflow uniformity, and cleanliness of the materials of construction. All these design parameters except material cleanliness are interrelated. Optimum filter design aims to balance these variables. Cleanliness of materials of construction is a relatively new requirement for cleanoom filters and is driven by increasing concerns for air borne molecular contamination.

The media is subject to a battery of tests during and after manufacture to check for conformity with specifications, efficiency and physical properties. After it is fabricated into a filter element in a rigid frame, further testing is done at the fabricator's workshop. Here the filters are graded according to the type of testing that is carried out.

Type A filters are subject to a routine efficiency/penetration test with challenge aerosol at 100% of prescribed concentration and airflow at 100% of rated capacity, using the total recovery method to check that overall penetration is below the acceptable limit.

Type B filters are challenged with 100% as well as 20% concentration/ airflow levels to check whether aggregate penetration remains proportional or varies inversely with flow rate.

If there are pinhole leaks in the media, penetration will increase with decreasing airflow, relatively independent of particle size. This is because the constriction of airflow through a pinhole is a function of the air velocity whenever the constriction of airflow through the fibrous filter media. Therefore, at 20% or one-fifth of full test flow, a pinhole shows up as 5 times greater in proportion to total flow than it does at full flow. Also, at higher velocities particles impact upon the fibres of the filter element directly, whereas at lower velocities Brownian motion causes them to drift and wander. In the process they are more likely to find their way out of the leak.

Another reason is that as airflow reduces, the leakage of the challenge aerosol through the pinhole causes an increases in the concentration downstream. The "masking" effect caused by surrounding "clean" airstreams is less pronounced.

Type C filter is not only tested for efficiency, but also *scanned* individually for pinhole leaks. When the filter element is installed at site, the only meaningful testing that can be carried out is a probe for gross leakage through gaskets or ruptures in the media.

Electrostatic and intermolecular forces play a keen role with ultrafines (particles smaller than 0.3 micron). These are usually charged particles that attract or repel other charged particles. When they attract, they coalesce and

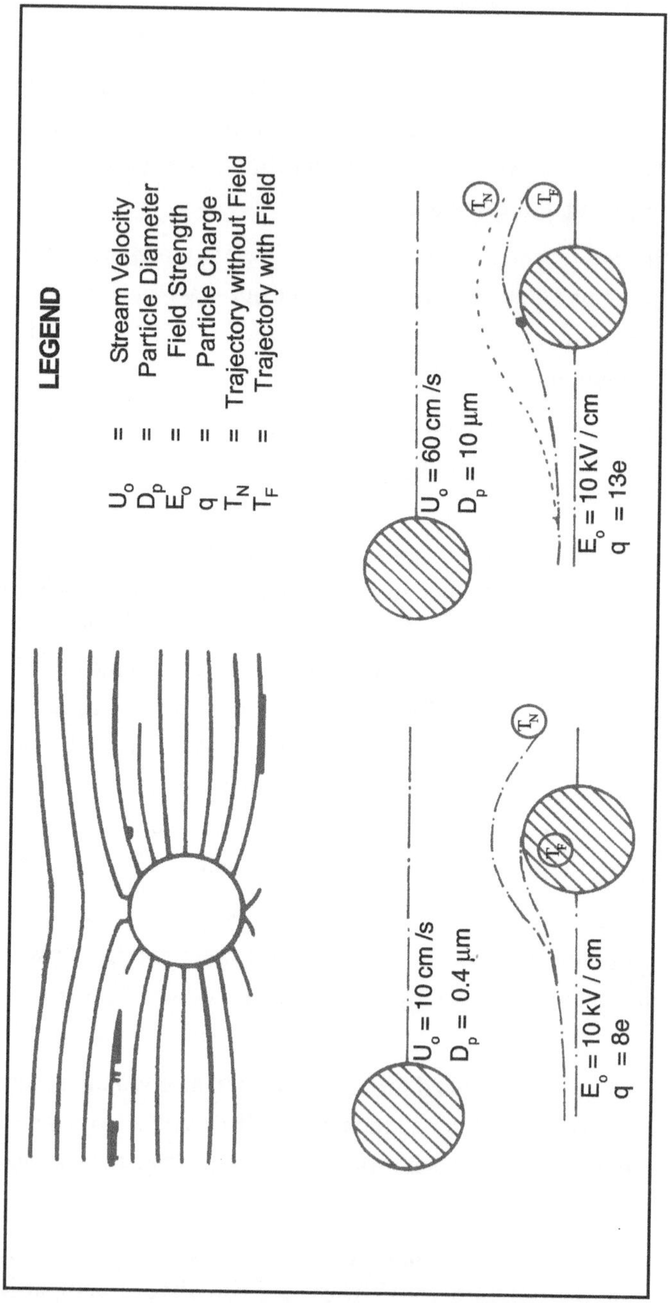

Figure 4.19 : Particle trajectories with and without an applied electric field

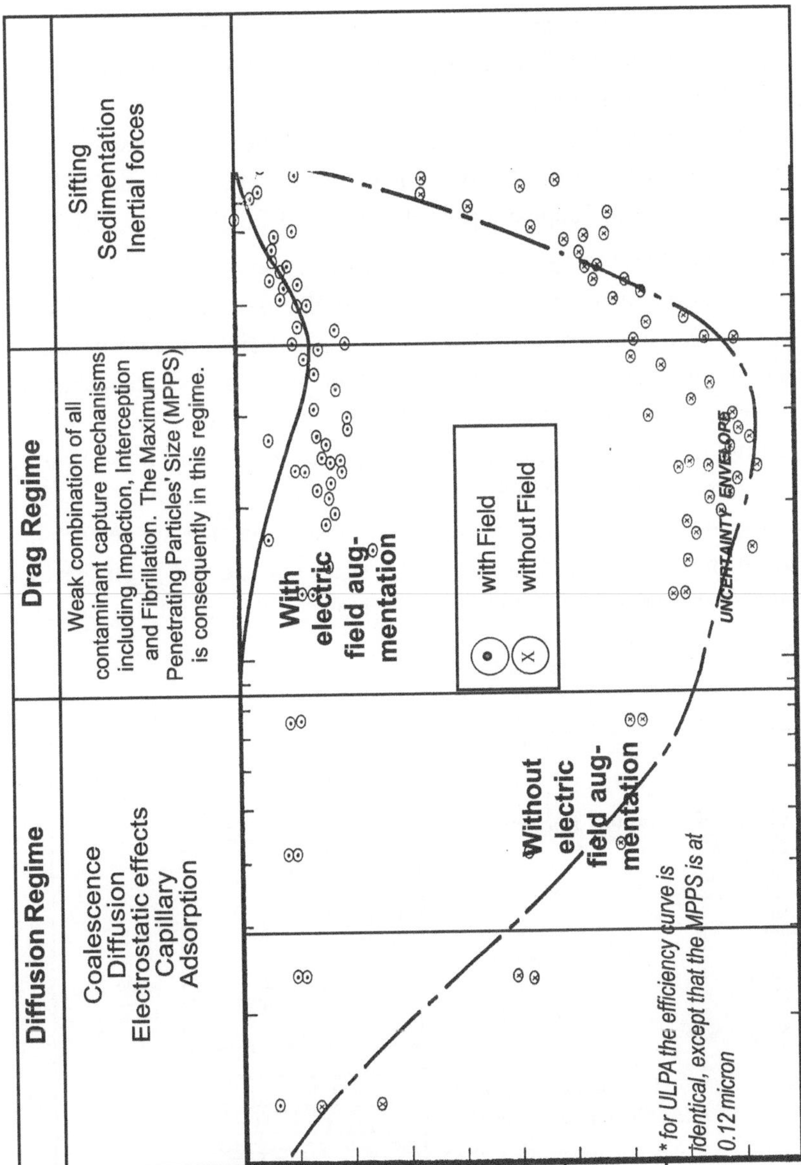

Figure 4.20 : HEPA Filtration Efficiency with & without Electric Field

agglomerate and grow into larger particles. (Most of the fine dust we encounter in cleanrooms despite rigorous cleaning regimen is proof of this phenomenon).

It is possible to improve the overall efficiency if we were to use a hybrid system that features electric field augmentation of HEPA/ULPA filtration. The presence of a group of dielectric fibres in an otherwise undisturbed electric field causes the lines of constant electric force to become distorted. The electric field polarizes the fibres, and charged particles will be attracted to the side of the fibre that is of opposite polarity to that of the particle.

In the process of charged particulates adhering to oppositely charged fibres, there is an interesting phenomenon that proves wholly to our advantage. Under normal circumstances where there is no such electric field, the accumulates smear on to the incident surface and block out the air pathways, thus choking up the filter. In stark contrast, the particulates captured by the polarised fibres accumulate on the incident face develop a dendritic formation leading to a strong lattice network which bonds well with the filter and acts as a physical extension of it. The lattice work permits airflow, thereby performing as an add-on prefilter. The dendritic effect is an unexpected boon that not only improves filtration efficiency with increasing dust build-up, but also

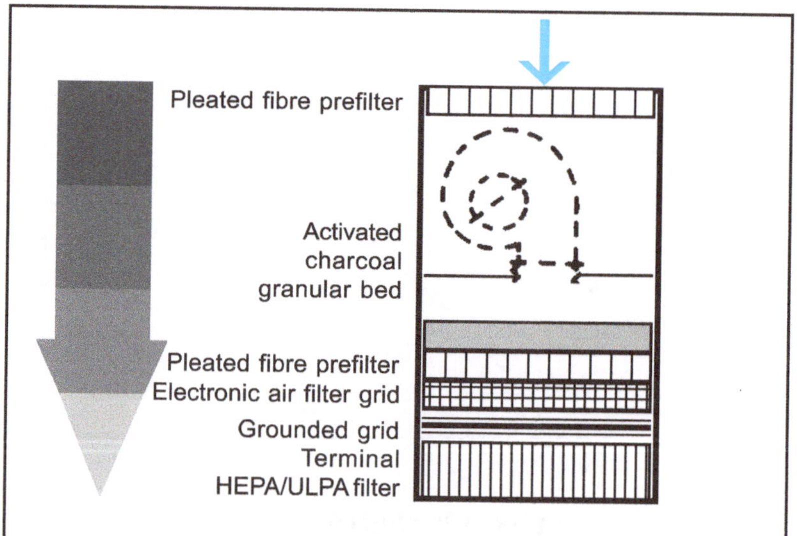

Fig. 4.21 A composite hybrid air filter assembly

extends the useful life of the terminal filter simultaneously. HEPA/ULPA filters featuring "Electrically Enhanced Filtration" (EEF) are commercially available.

A comprehensive hybrid filtration system includes prefiltration with a coarser (and less expensive) pleated filter, chemical filter, an intermediate electronic filter and terminal or final HEPA/ULPA filter. This filter configuration exhibits improved filtration efficiency across the suspended contaminant size range, markedly in the MPPS regime.

Before we close our discussion of air filters, here are some recommendations the User of HEPA filters should consider:

Filter size vs structural rigidity: Experience indicates that single filters featuring separators having a depth less than 25% of the smaller side dimension may not be able to meet the pressure handling requirements; larger sizes may present significant problems in handling and have doubtful mechanical stability. In separatorless type construction, filter depth in excess of the prescribed 69.9 mm (2.75") may compromise rigidity of the pack.

Filter pleats: In applications where filter faces are mounted vertically (horizontal laminar airflow work station, for example), pleats and separators should be vertical. Sagging of pack may occur if filters are installed with separators horizontal, which may result in media failure or uneven flow conditions. The filter medium supports should not vary from a straight line by more than 6.4 mm (0.25"), and crest to crest contacts on adjacent folds should not vary by more than 1.6 mm (0.0625").

Number of pleats x Media Area per pleat x 5 fpm = Rated Capacity

Filter patching: The patching of tears, leaks and pinholes in filter media is a common manufacturing practice. The patch area should not exceed 13 cm^2 (2 sq inches)in any one spot or exceed a total of 1% of the area of the filter face. Spot patching with media or adhesive causes some velocity reduction in the vicinity, but may not normally detract from performance. In elevated temperature applications or those involving hazardous materials, the pressure of local patches may cause overheating and subsequent failure in that location.

Dead spots: The splicing or patching of filter media within the interior of the pleated pack may create local points of high resistance that impede flow resulting in areas of extremely low velocity (dead spots) in comparison to average velocity. Such conditions may be detrimental to laminar airflow work station performance.

Torn or bent separators: The presence of torn, crushed or bent separators in a filter may or may not be indicative of media damage. Where such conditions exist it is advisable to conduct a careful visual inspection (with filters illuminated from the rear side) ascertain whether media or sealant crack has occurred. If still in doubt, scan for leaks using cold DOP aerosol challenge.

5 Laminar Airflow

Laminar (or *unidirectional*) airflow as applied to industrial cleanroom technology is defined as airflow in which the entire mass of air within a confined space moves with uniform velocity along parallel (or non-intersecting) flow lines. The credit for development of this technique for airborne contamination control is generally attributed to Whitfield of Sandia Corporation, USA, who termed it as "a piston of clean air" pushing out suspended contaminants from the work environment.

In practice, achievement of *true* laminar airflow, as defined above, is never possible. A suspended particle in space can move in any direction - forward or backward; leftward or rightward; upward or downward. However, when entrained in a laminar air stream, it moves *predominantly in one direction*. In other words, its velocity along the direction of airflow is substantially larger than any component of velocity in any other direction. If the direction of flow is along the X-axis and the velocity is U, then

$$U_x \gg U_y, \; U_z$$

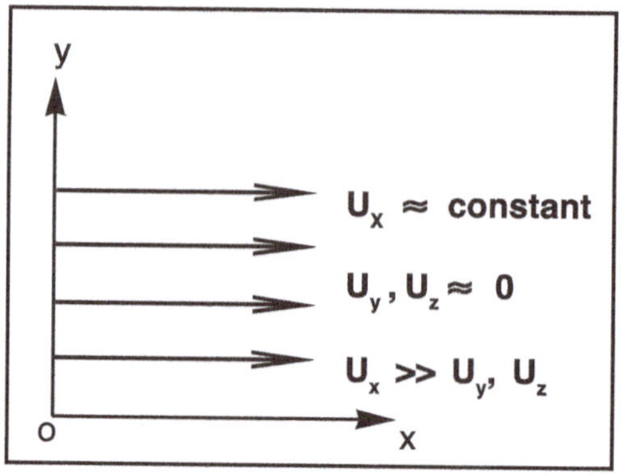

Fig. 5.1 Unidirectional laminar airflow

Besides, true *parallel* flow is precluded by the practical necessity of placing objects (including people) within the confined space. Although any object so placed will cause discontinuities in the flow pattern, these disturbed areas are swept out by the continuous flow of clean air.

Furthermore, air patterns tend to reestablish themselves within a distance approximately equal to three to five times the equivalent diameter of the object. The region immediately downstream of the obstructing object, known as the *wake* zone, is at relatively low pressure (*Bernoulli effect*), with strong turbulent currents, whose intensity decreases as we near the point in space where the air pattern returns to normal. This entire zone of low pressure is known as the *cone of turbulence*, where the apex of the cone is at an approximate distance of 3 to 5 times the equivalent diameter from the obstructing object (forming the base of the cone).

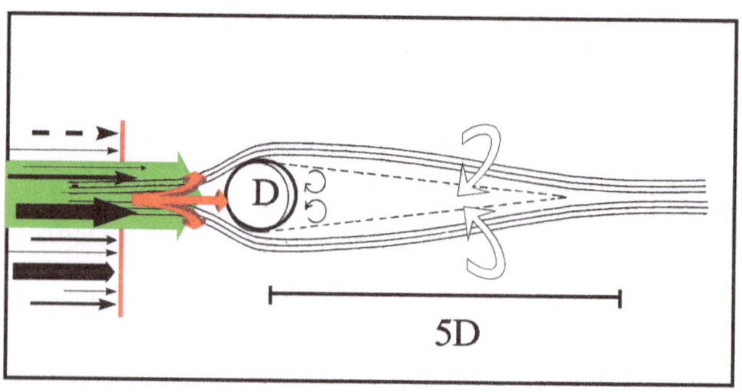

Fig. 5.2 Wake region disturbance & cone of turbulence

Air velocity in the laminar range is determined by Reynold's Number (N).

$$N = \rho UD/\mu$$

where ρ is the fluid density, U is the flow speed, D is a characteristic length and μ is the fluid viscosity.
Since both ρ and μ are functions of temperature, the velocity range in the laminar regime will vary with temperature too.
In typical cleanroom conditions, the mean value is 0.5 mps (100 fpm) with a standard deviation of 0.065 mps (13 fpm), which translates to a total range of 0.305 (61 fpm) to 0.695 mps (139 fpm). The ISO Standards allow down to 0.2 mps (40 fpm); but the Orange Guide 2002 still insists on 0.45 mps +/- 0.1 mps (90 +/- 20 fpm).

Behind each product or work piece placed in clean laminar airflow there is such a cone; if the apex of the cone lies well inside the clean space, the turbulent air, being clean, will not jeopardise the product; but if part of the cone extends to contaminated space, the low pressures in the wake will aspirate the contaminated air and increase the risk of product contamination.

Suspended contaminants present in air when a laminar airflow system is first turned on are propelled out of the cleanroom or work space in the first pass, clearance being typically obtained within a few minutes due to the high rate of air exchange, and at steady state the suspended contaminant density is largely determined by that generated within the room.

The air velocity in industrial laminar airflow installations is 0.3 to 0.6 mps (60 - 120 fpm), which is almost imperceptible, much less than

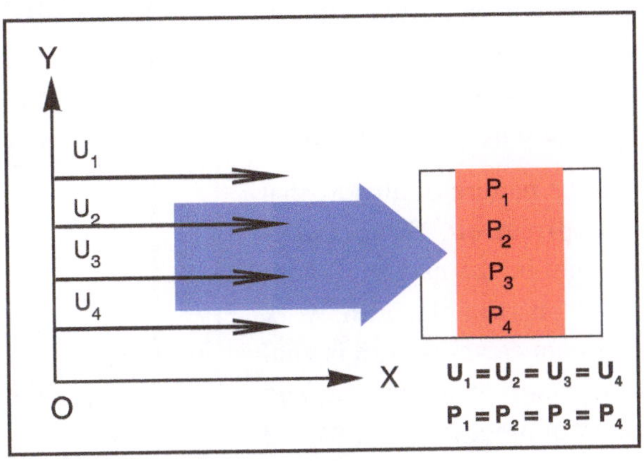

Fig. 5.3

the force felt when walking at one mile per hour on a still day. Although this velocity is very low, it is much higher than the rate at which suspended particles tend to settle. For example, a 10μ sand particle falls in still air at 1.5 fpm, and a bacteria (1μ) at less than an inch per minute.

In other words, if the 10μ sand particle were dropped in an industrial horizontal laminar airflow installation, it would travel 20' horizontally along direction of airflow while dropping less than 4" vertically. The bacteria would have dropped less than a quarter of an inch over the same distance. Laminar airflow, therefore, gives little opportunity to the suspended contaminants it encounters to settle down and moves them out along predetermined flow lines, away from vulnerable sites, passing any point in space lying in its path once, and only once. If the suspended contaminant, entrained upstream of the product, passes a critical site without impinging or settling, it will never return to that site again. In contrast, in turbulent airflow, the eddy currents present can, and often do, allow a contaminant to return again and again.

However, the cost of a laminar airflow room is prohibitive, and most designers rely on localised laminar airflow work stations at critical work sites to protect against aerial contamination, and opt for the more economical mixed flow or turbulent flow cleanrooms, where filtered air is dispersed at multiple-terminals scattered in the ceiling.

Laminar airflow workstations are used for either or both of the following:

Product protection for operations involving materials that must be kept sterile or free from unwanted ecological agents; and *agent containment* for manipulations involving etiological agents, materials or procedures requiring personnel protection, where the items in use must be confined within the working area and not allowed to escape into the environment.

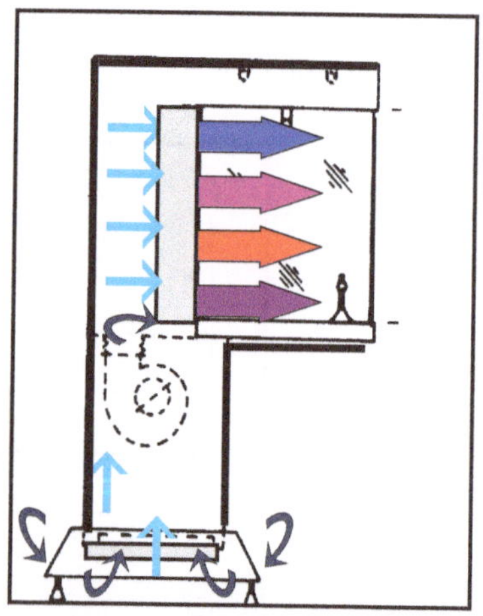

Fig. 5.4 Horizontal laminar flow clean air work station

For selecting the pattern of airflow that best suits an application, the primary consideration would be the nature of work being carried out on the clean air work station. For optimum cleanliness, it is vital that the flow of clean air across, on and around the product or process be maintained at a maximum.

Horizontal flow systems offer maximum product protection, and are, by far, the most effective form of contamination control. They call for the least in operator discipline where the work activity involves physical manipulation. Operators may bend their heads, or other parts of their bodies over or around the work site without seriously jeopardising it. The work table edge is deemed to be the boundary separating the clean space from the contaminated environment, and care must be taken to ensure that the apex of any cone of turbulence generated in the clean space does not penetrate this boundary. These systems, however, are unsuitable for operations where toxic fumes or vapours are encountered, or for work with open vessels of chemicals, solvents or powders, since horizontal flow would raise vapour levels in the room, increase solvent drag-out and distribute powder particles throughout the environment, resulting in not only greater contamination levels within, but also enhanced risks of cross contamination through operators who may be moving from station to station.

In some cases, the production equipment bulk may preclude parallel horizontal flow across the work surface and cause eddies which could negate the very purpose of a clean air bench. For such and other similar applications, specially involving agent containment, a vertical downward airflow configuration is more appropriate. Vertical downflow is also favoured for procedures that do not require eye-hand coordination, and for equipment which is semiautomatic or fully-automatic.

Horizontal LF systems are generally fitted with a protective grille downstream of the HEPA filter to prevent accidental damage to the media as well as to serve as a secondary plenum for pressure stabilisation. Unfortunately, fine particles that penetrate the filter often impact on this grille, and over a period of time a film or coating builds up behind this grille, leading to the hazard of intermittent emissions caused by mechanical vibration or sudden variations in airflow. (Had the fine particles not been arrested, in all probability they may have just floated past the work site; but the agglomeration on the incident face of the protective grille coughs up much larger sized particles whose contaminating potential is much enhanced.)

Unlike Horizontal LF, where airflow is unobstructed, the vertical downward flow impinges directly on the work surface, which marks a dead-end. Perforations on the work surface improves matters somewhat, but it is still far from adequate. In the process, an envelope of air cushion builds up over

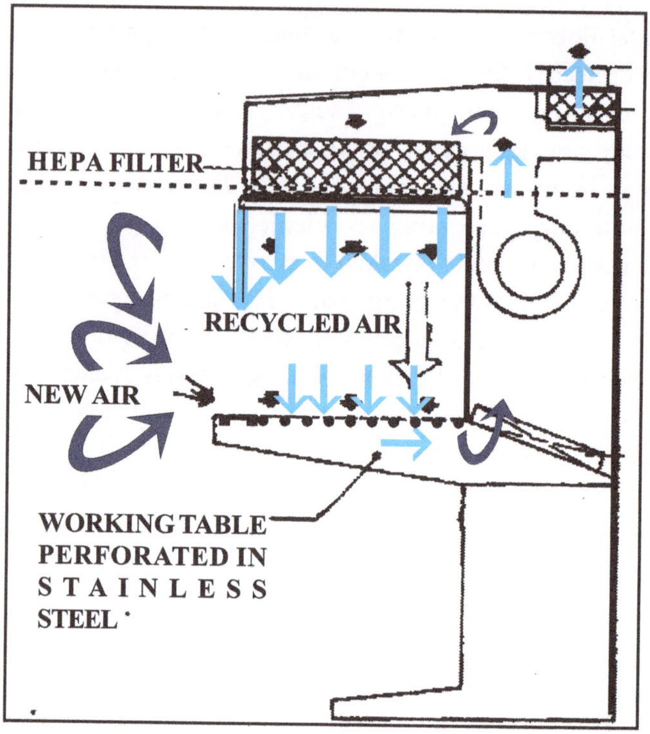

Fig. 5. 5 Vertical laminar downflow clean air work station

the surface, causing clean air entering the work space to deviate towards the work station exit face much before it reaches the work surface. Designs that feature partial or total exhaust, however, have a better control over the airflow distribution within the work space. Among the innovations in this design is the partial recirculatory system, which sucks back up to 60% of the air from the work space through return ducts terminating in slots along the periphery of the work surface.

Whenever work space air is exhausted from the room, there is partial negative pressure with respect to the room at the work space. To prevent room air from contaminating the product, designs provide for an air curtain (high velocity sheath of air) along the entry face with perforations on the work table edge, so that the air ingress is out of harm's way. Unlike fume exhaust chambers, clean air LF work stations do not allow makeup air into the main work area. The table edge, for example, is generally made to protrude outward slightly, so that the perforations on the surface to draw in the makeup air is marginally outside the plane of the air barrier.

Room air, being filtered and tempered, is too expensive to be cast out as exhaust indiscriminately. To minimise the quantum so exhausted, a design innovation termed *add-air*, or auxiliary air feed system, is commonly employed, whereby a controlled amount of untempered air from outside the clean environment (usually a corridor) is drawn in to complement the air sucked in from the room. In this process, the exhaust volume requirements are met; the work space is contained under negative pressure; the product site is protected; and only the bare minimum quantity of room air is used up.

Many design innovations in the laminar airflow pattern have been introduced. Instead of having a piston of air moving with the same constant velocity, the velocity profile could be graded, such that adjacent streams are at marginally differing velocities, while retaining the entire mass within acceptable LF limits (vary from 60 fpm to 120 fpm). This yields superior airstream integrity, specially while confronting obstructing objects.

Air could be made to converge or focus on the work site for enhanced dilution and cleandown. Likewise, it could be diverging to spread clean air and extend the clean zone perimeter. While the latter two have air streams that are not parallel, their velocity is within the laminar range.

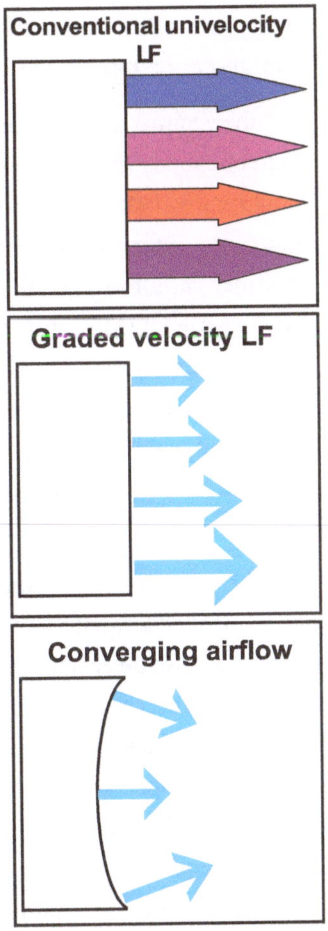

Fig. 5. 6 Laminar flow variations

Radial airflow allows effective utilisation of floor space by accommodating several operators at the work table who do not get into each other's way. Inclined airflow permits bringing the object or equipment to be protected much closer to the filter.

In certain cases of containment, the product aerosols must be kept away from the operator. Powder weighing and dispensing is a common application. To guarantee such protection by isolation, reverse laminar airflow techniques are employed.

The plenum is maintained under negative pressure in some patented designs, such that if a filter is ill-fitted or develops a leak in its gasket, clean air from the work space is sucked back through the gap in the filter seating, rather than allow unfiltered air to bypass the filter and contaminate the work space.

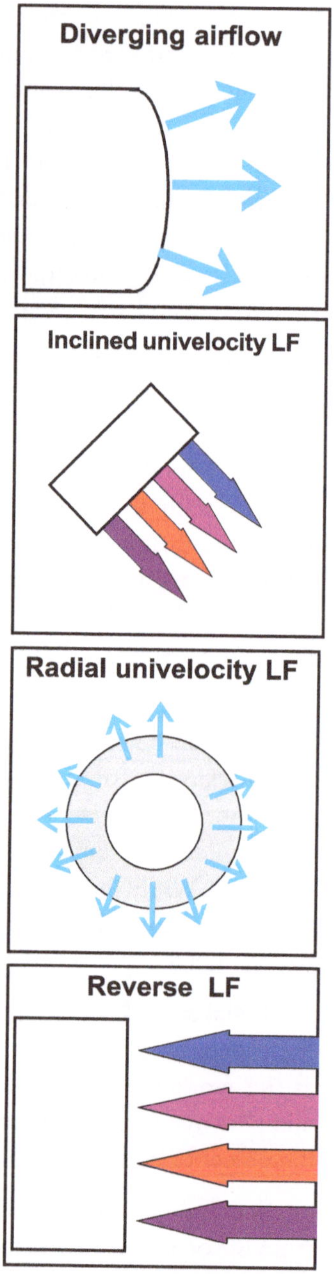

Fig. 5. 7 More laminar flow variations

Other improvements include incorporation of chemical adsorbent filters for vapour, gas and odour removal; desiccants for moisture removal; electronic intermediate filters for enhanced ultrafines capture and static control; multispeed and variable speed motor-blowers or the more recent "smart" motor-blower that automatically adjusts speed to compensate for filter loading; and chilled water line complete with thermostat and humidistat for temperature and humidity control.

Other improvements include incorporation of chemical adsorbent filters for vapour, gas and odour removal; desiccants for moisture removal; electronic intermediate filters for enhanced ultrafines capture and static control; multispeed and variable speed motor-blowers or the more recent "smart" motor-blower that automatically adjusts speed to compensate for filter loading; and chilled water line complete with thermostat and humidistat for temperature and humidity control.

The question of choice of material for bulkhead execution is often asked, and the answer is coloured by the camp answering. In practice, it does not really matter as long as the construction is rugged, has a cleanroom grade

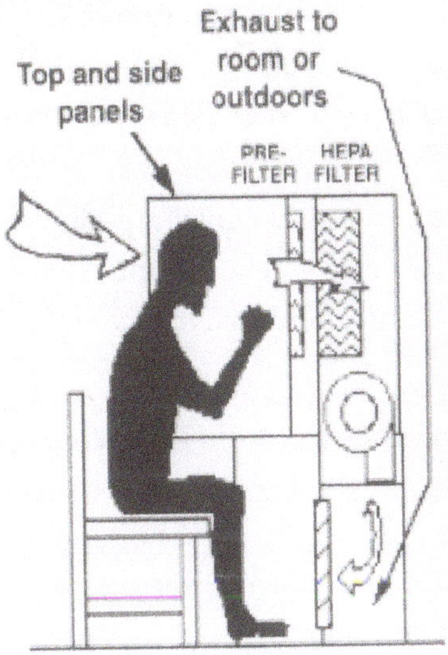

Fig. 5. 8 Reverse laminar flow work station

surface finish, can withstand normal rigours of cleanroom sanitation chemicals and damps noise and vibration to acceptable levels.

In some designs, like a clean air tent, the sides are often enclosed with panels, While such panels help isolate the interior, the boundary layer separation of airflow at the periphery causes aspiration of outside air into the enclosure (Bernoulli effect). If the design features an integral clean air barrier all along the inner perimeter, such invading aerosols can be contained.

Laminar airflow guarantees stability in the parametric profiles (temperature, humidity contaminant density and air velocity) along its path. At the point where this ceases to be the case, laminarity may be deemed to be lost.

Before we close, let us emphasise that laminarity relates to air *velocity* and not to air *cleanliness*. We can have turbulent air which is Class 100 clean; and true laminar airflow of unclean air. To make double sure that we want both, we say Class 100 Laminar Airflow.

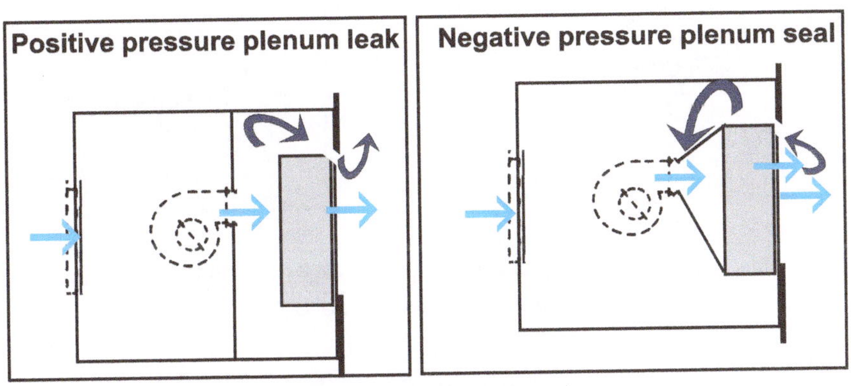

Fig. 5. 9 HEPA sealing

Another advantage arising from such unidirectional non-turbulent streamline flow at uniform velocity is that parametric gradients are not disturbed. They remain stable. The points in space with identical parametric values are referred to as being isoparametric. For example, points in space with identical contaminant density, or number of particles per unit volume, are known as isopleths. Laminar airflow may be relied upon to guarantee stable isopleths. As a corollary, when isopleths cease to be stable, laminar airflow ceases to exist.

Here are interesting inputs on unidirectional airflow from ISO 14644-4:

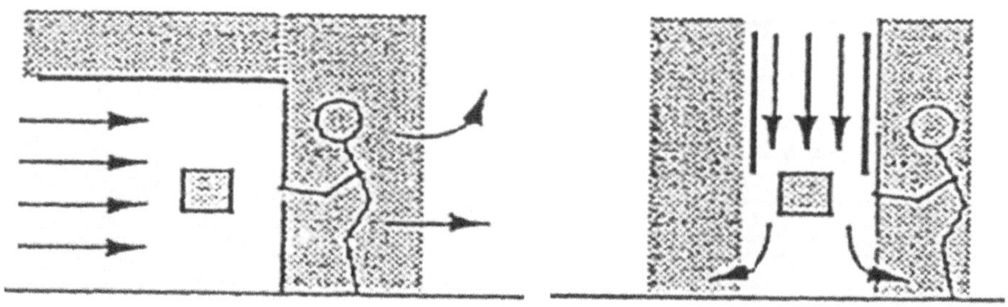

Fig. 5. 10: Product protection

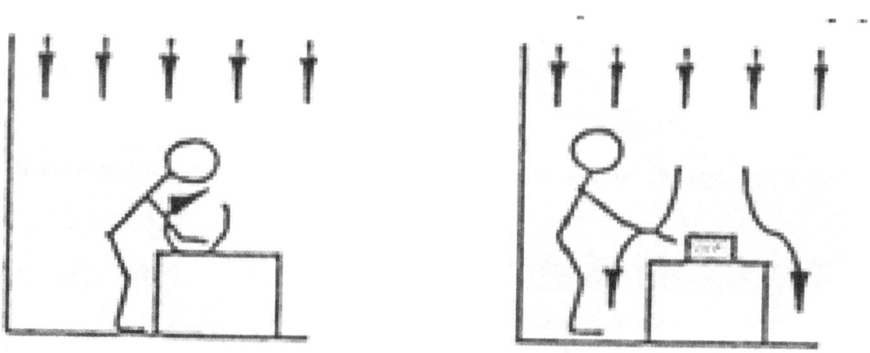

Fig. 5. 11: Disturbance of unidirectional airflow
Improvement by personnel behaviour

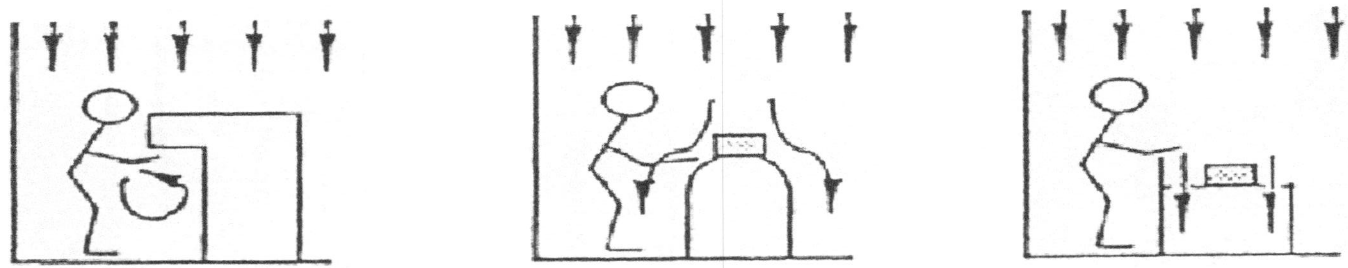

Fig. 5. 12: Disturbance of unidirectional airflow
Improvement by personnel behaviour

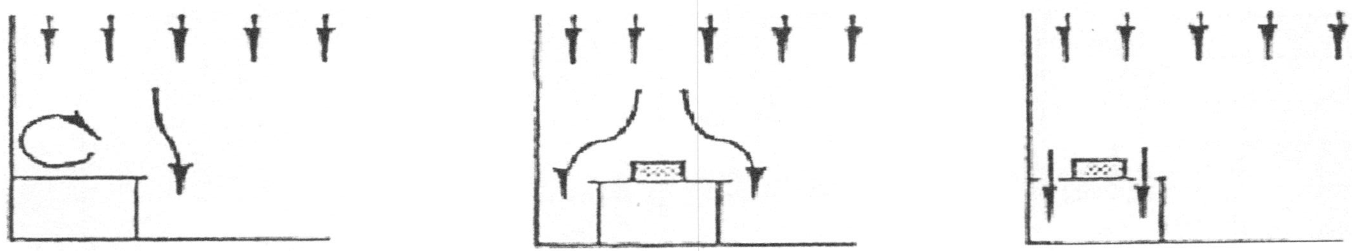

Fig. 5. 13: Disturbance of unidirectional airflow
Improvement by arrangement

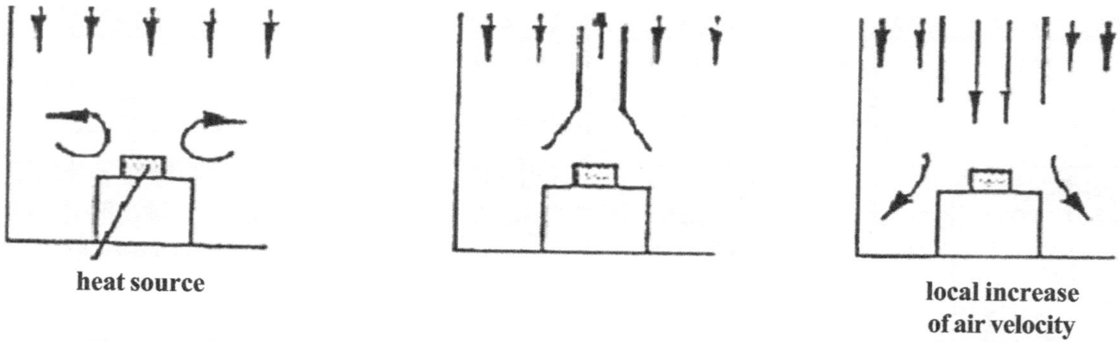

Fig. 5. 14: Disturbance of unidirectional airflow Improvement by airflow concept

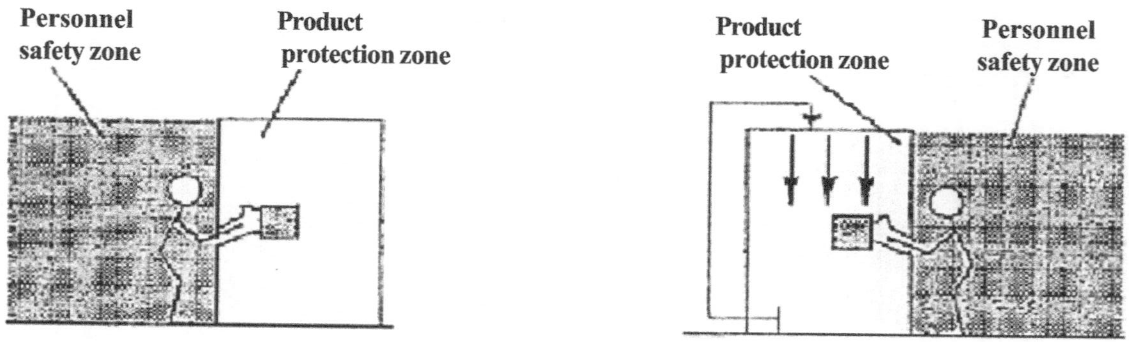

Fig. 5. 15: Passive & Active Systems

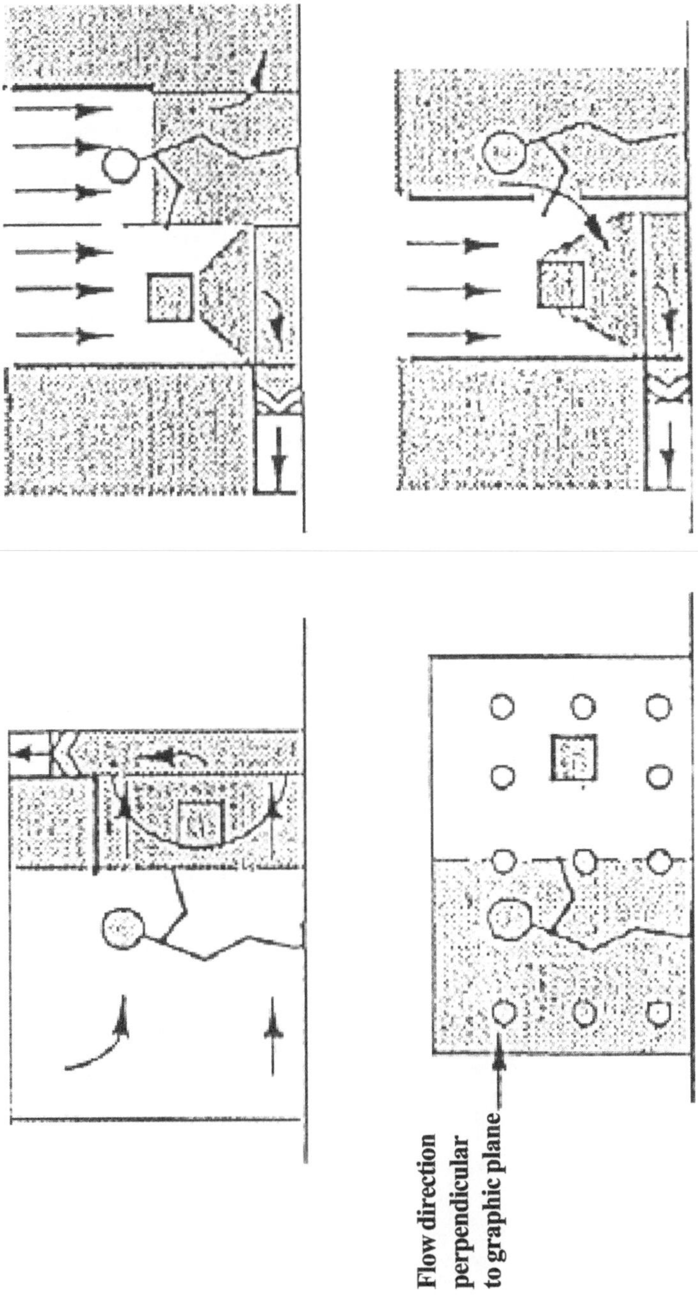

Fig. 5. 16: Personnel/environment/product protection

6 Qualification

Qualification is a process of testing and verification. This term has now been extended to encompass checking that an element or equipment conforms to previously agreed specifications (DQ); that it has been installed correctly (IQ or *as built*); it operates as expected (OQ or *at rest*), and plays its designated role satisfactorily when the facility is fully functional (FQ or *operational*). As opposed to *validation*, where the focus is on a particular *method, process or procedure* that, if carried out as prescribed, will guarantee a desired result, qualification is more restrictive in that it is confined to checking out a particular aspect for conformity.

A filter or clean environment is *qualified*; not *validated*. But the Standard Operating Procedure (SOP) for performing qualification must be *validated*.

One of the elements in your contamination control programme is your cleanroom, where several parameters need to be verified. Procedures must be established for qualification for acceptance as well as qualification for proving continued compliance.

Qualification should be the responsibility of a *task team* with members drawn from Production, Engineering, QA and Microbiology; and this team should coordinate with any external contracting agency that may be involved in the execution of some or all of the tests.

Qualification could be episodic; routine; continual or continuous. Not all parameters can or need be checked continuously. For example, air filter integrity or illumination; but some critical parameters can vary so widely and quickly that intermittent sampling may not suffice. You need to be sure that the environment continues to operate within design limits *every minute of every day.* With increasing batch volumes in parenterals and decreasing line widths in microelectronics the consensus is toward continuous on-line monitoring of critical parameters. The Draft USFDA Guidelines for Aseptic Processing of Sterile Products, Orange Guide 2002 and ISO 14644-2: all recommend this practice.

Having said that, the results we obtain should be reliable, relevant and representative, based on which some action can be initiated. Data interpretation is as important, if not more, than data collection. If the data is incomplete, inaccurate or misleading, it will be more hindrance than help.

Some sample documents are reproduced at the end of this chapter to serve as references for drawing up your own programme.

We commence by examining the procedures for testing air filters, before moving on to testing and certifying cleanrooms and LAF devices.

Testing Prefilters

The complexities of filtration principles and the many varieties of aerosol filters can present a perplexing choice to the designer of a practical system. There is no single answer for testing or comparing filters under all application conditions or for the proper filter for a specific job. The rating of a filter is based on its resistance to airflow, its aerosol removal capabilities, and its dust holding capacity.

Rating standards for general ventilation or air-conditioning grade filters (used as *prefilters in cleanrooms*) are covered in ASHRAE Standard 52.1, which provides two measures of *removal* capability: *Arrestance*, a weight percentage removal rating based on tests with a synthetic dust, and *Atmospheric dust spot efficiency*, a percentage removal rating based on staining tests with normal atmospheric dust. *Dust holding capacity* is determined using synthetic dust.

Ratings may be expressed for clean conditions, or as averages over the dust holding capacity life of the filter. Thus in interpreting filter test data it is important to realise that they provide a comparison of different filter types, and that the actual performance in any one application may differ significantly from the test results.

Arrestance or weight efficiency test: This test is based on an artificial dust mixture consisting of 72% standardised air cleaner test dust, fine: 23% Molocco black, and 5% of #7 cotton linters ground in a Wilney mill with a 4 mm screen, all percentages by weight. A known amount of dust is introduced upstream of the filter under test, and the dust penetrating the filter is collected and weighed to give a measure of efficiency. It must be borne in mind, however, that in any normal air sample, though the bigger particles are fewer than the smaller particles, they represent a larger proportion of the total weight. The remaining weight of smaller particles represents a very large number. Thus a high gravimetric arrestance percentage by this technique does not necessarily indicate a high removal capability for the smaller particles of concern for most applications.

Atmospheric dust spot efficiency test: On the other hand, does reflect the effect of smaller particles, with the challenge aerosol being the naturally occurring dust in the environment. The optical densities of filter paper samples upstream and downstream of the filter under evaluation are compared to produce a rating of the dust's staining abilities after filtration. Since smaller particles cause staining more readily, this technique is more indicative of small particle removal and less sensitive to large particle penetration.

Dust holding capacity: Is an accelerated life test based on synthetic dust, and is usually performed concurrently with *arrestance* and *dust spot efficiency* tests. Dust holding capacity is defined as the amount of dust fed to the filter *times* its average arrestance during test to the point of maximum rated resistance, or to the point where arrestance falls to 85% - 75% of maximum.

It is readily apparent that each of the filter test standards is biased in one form or another, and any extrapolation beyond their intended range of applicability is questionable. Claims of efficiency are meaningless, unless the corresponding test method is specified. For example, a typical prefilter has a 99% weight efficiency, 83% dust spot efficiency and 55% DOP efficiency.

Testing HEPAs and ULPAs

At the media manufacturers' end, testing a HEPA or ULPA includes visual inspection for imperfections and mechanical measurement of media parameters, apart from filtration efficiency. Basis weight is checked on a Basis Weight Scale; thickness by an automatic micrometer; tensile strength, both in machine direction and cross-machine direction; stiffness; percent combustibles; water repellency; Frazier porosity and pressure drop. However, the User's interest is restricted to tests on the filter after it has been fabricated: the efficiency, integrity, airflow capacity and pressure drop of the fabricated assembly. Components of filters in microelectronics are increasingly being tested for off gassing of molecular contaminants such as boron, phosphor and organic compounds.

While ASHRAE tests, being destructive, are made on a sample basis, which assumes that the filter being tested is representative of the product, the tests for HEPA and ULPA grades are nondestructive procedures, designed to permit 100% inspection. The limitation, of course, is that these results relate to monodisperse aerosol behaviour only.

Table 6.1: Current aerosol challenge materials for HEPA and ULPA filter testing

Standard or Recommended Practice	Country	Material	Aerosol and its detection Avg. size µm	Detection η% ΔP	Leak limits
IES-RP-CC001.3-93	USA	DOP	0.30	Area/ Qty	
IES-RP-CC007 1-92	USA	DOP	0.18	Qty	-
DIN 24184	D	Paraffin	0.45	Area	
EUROVENT 4/4	Europe	NaCl	0.60	Mass	-
BS 3928	GB	NaCl	0.60	Mass	-
AFNOR X 44013	F	NaCl	0.60	Mass	-
AFNOR X 41011	F	Uranine	0.15	Mass	-
prEN 1822 (1995)	Europe	DEHS	MPPS	Qty	

Table 6.2 : Properties of challenge aerosols

Material	Ref. Std.	Gravimetric Concentration µg / litre	Photometric Concentration Readings %
DOP/DEHP	US IES-RP	102.0	100.0
DOS/DEHS	CEN EN 1822	77.7	82.0
PEG 400		67.1	56.0
Emery 3004	US FDA	85.0	112.0
BP ENERPAR M-00	German DIN 28124	79.4	90.0

HEPA and ULPA grade filtration performance rating is covered by US Mil Standards 282, F-51477 (Fire resistant) or F-51068 (Fire retardant) and the AACC Standard CS-1T. These should be read in conjunction with IES-RP-CC-001/ 2/6/7/34, and others adopted in Europe, which provide procedures for determining removal efficiency based on penetration tests with artificially produced monodisperse aerosols of submicronic size at rated airflow and rated pressure drop. These rating tests are not necessarily relevant to actual particle laden environments with particle size distributions different from those used for the tests.

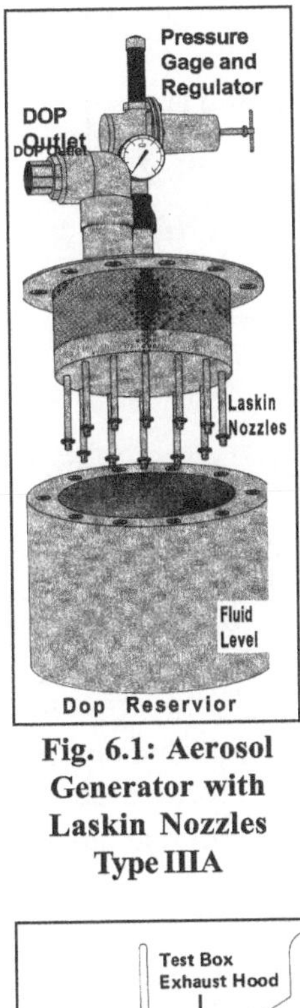

Fig. 6.1: Aerosol Generator with Laskin Nozzles Type IIIA

Filter efficiency test: This test is carried out by the filter manufacturer at his factory using a monodisperse challenge. The total filter is challenged at one time and a single reading of penetration is obtained.

The Efficiency of a filter is determined by measuring the challenge aerosol concentration up and downstream of a filter. Then,

Efficiency = 1 – (Downstream Concentration / Upstream Concentration)

Opinions are sharply divided with regard to the best test method for assessing the efficiency of HEPAs or ULPAs. The British employ sodium chloride (salt spray and hydrogen flame - sodium flame photometric test); the French use Uranine dyes; the Germans prefer paraffin oil; the Russians work with optical microscopes and densitometers; and the Americans abide by aerosols and mass photometry.

The most commonly used test procedure in USA and

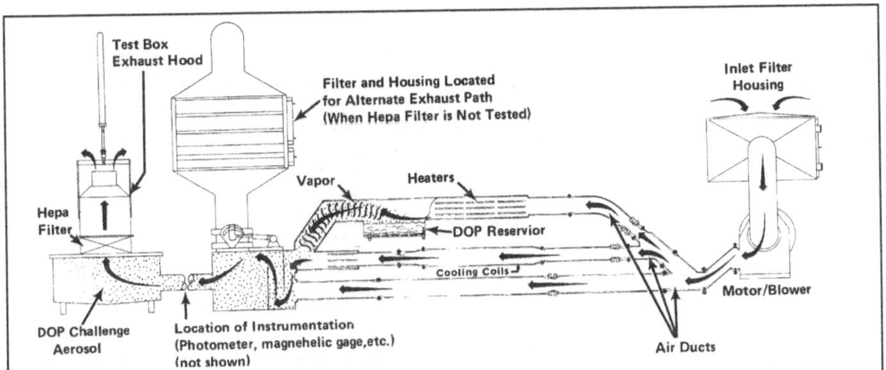

Fig. 6.2: HEPA filter efficiency testing using thermally generated DOP

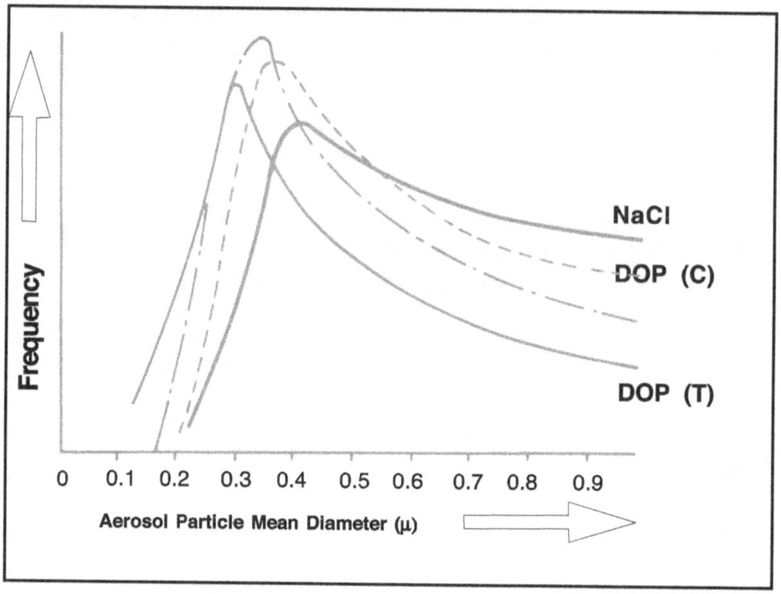

Fig. 6.3: Droplet size distributions of aerosols

India is the penetrometer technique using Di-Octyl-Pthalate (DOP) oil, or, to be more exact, DEHP (Di-2 ethyl-hexyl-pthalate), which is atomised by a special nozzle to produce an aerosol. Type IIIA Laskin nozzle delivers DOP vapour at a concentration of 5.1 mg/litre. This is diluted to 100 μg/litre by mixing with 3.82 m^3/min (135 cfm) of clean air per nozzle. When cold DOP is atomised through Laskin nozzles, a polydispersed aerosol is obtained, with particle size in the range of 0.45μ to 3.0μ, with median size at 0.72μ. For filter efficiency testing a polydisperse aerosol will not do. Fortunately, hot DOP smoke has a very narrow, uniform, controlled particle size, which can be increased or decreased by varying the temperature. To attain and sustain 0.3μ particle size, the temperature is maintained at 72 ^{0}F.

Table 6.2: Count Vs Mass median diameters of Cold and Thermal DOP

Aerosol	Concentration* μg / litre of air	μm CMD	μm MMD	Correction factor
Cold DOP	~30	0.25	0.69	1.00
Thermal DOP	18	0.25	0.50	1.00

CMD : Count Median Diameter

MMD : Mass Median Diameter

* With 95% confidence limit based on 5 measurements for each liquid.

A sophisticated generator is used for carefully controlling oil and air temperature, airflow rate and mixing conditions to produce *hot* DOP smoke as a challenge aerosol. DOP oil is heated in a reservoir through which hot air at 365 °F is passed, causing the oil to evaporate and be carried forward in the hot air stream. The test rig is usually several meters long with multiple ducts fitted with mechanical baffles for removal of oversize and under-size droplets. This oil-air mixture is then quenched with cooler air maintained at 72 °F.

The particle concentration detector is typically a forward scattering photometer employing a white light bulb as the light source, and a sensitive photomultiplier tube as the detector. The photometer is first calibrated for zero with clean air flowing through the scattering chamber. Then it is calibrated for 100%, with DOP smoke filling the system. The percent penetration of a filter is measured by the amount of DOP smoke that gets through the media at a concentration of 100 mg/m^3 or 100 μgrams/litre at rated airflow for efficiency measurements, and at 20% of rated flow to probe for pinhole leaks. (As explained earlier, one of the characteristics of fibre filter media is that leakage through a pinhole is better detected at lower flow rates). At the same time, filter resistance at the test flow rate is measured.

State of the art in DOP type aerosol challenge features two special laser probes to simultaneously sample upstream and downstream of the filter. A

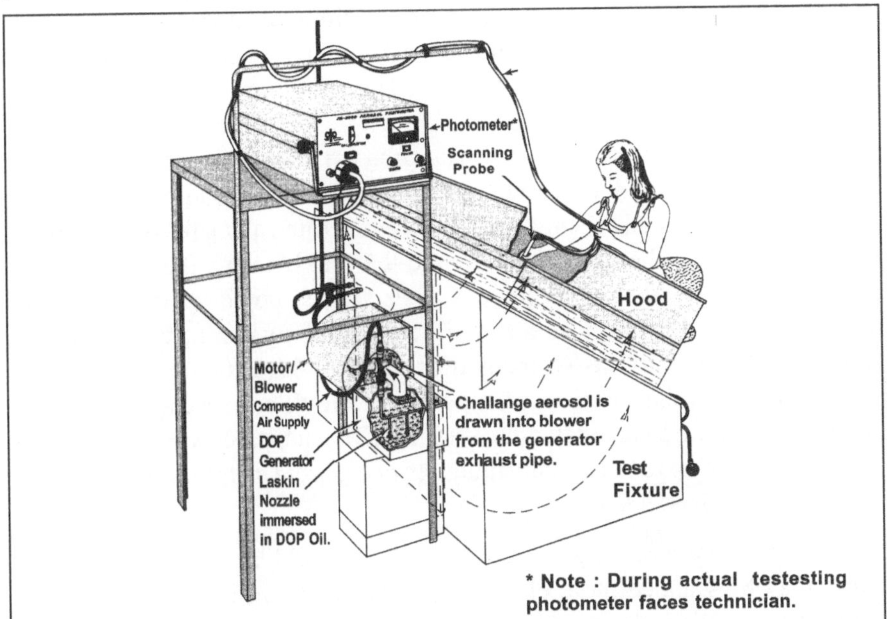

Fig. 6.4: Scanning HEPA filter for leaks

polydispersed cold DOP smoke generated within is neutralised with a K-85 radioactive source. The resulting aerosol is passed through the filter, and the information sensed by the probes is processed by a special laser aerosol photometer. This system can count particles according to 32 separate size ranges from 0.09μ to 3μ. The results are further computed and graphs of fractional efficiency are displayed or printed. These systems are routinely used to test for efficiency in the range 99.9999%.

Since a filter's efficiency increases as it accumulates particulate matter in service, the initial efficiency is the lowest efficiency in the life of that filter. Minute areas of greater penetration, either in the edge sealant between the filter element and the filter's integral rigid frame, or in the filter element itself, are often present, but when the filter is tested these are diluted by the greater amount of air passing through the filter. Such deficiencies can be tolerated as long as the overall penetration through the filter does not exceed prescribed limits.

Scanning for leaks in installed filters at site: In-place field test of an installed filter does not measure its *efficiency*, and should not be so considered. This test is made with a polydispersed challenge, which only reveals the presence of leaks, if any, in the installation.

When a filter under test is accessible, probing for leaks is relatively easy and straight forward. Cold DOP is atomised through Laskin nozzles, and a polydispersed aerosol is obtained, with particle size in the range of 0.45μ to 3.0μ, with median size at 0.72μ. The sampling probe is held into the airflow at a distance of 25mm (1") from the filter face and scanned by passing the probe in slightly overlapping strokes at a traverse rate of 3 m/min (10 fpm), so that the entire face of the filter is sampled. Separate passes are made around the entire periphery of the filter, along the bond between the filter pack and the frame, and around the seal between the filter and the device. If any sudden or suspicious deflection is noted on the meter, the probe is returned to the location and held stationary for further sampling, since the sensitivity to leaks is many times higher with a stationary probe than with a moving probe. Prolonged exposure of the filter to the aerosol should be avoided. If a HEPA is rated for 99.97% efficiency, a downstream aerosol concentration of up to 0.03% constitutes an *acceptable penetration*, any higher value being deemed a *leak*

Since filters are rectangular, the probe too should be rectangular, so that edges may be scanned more effectively. The sampling rate is 1 CFM. For isokinetic sampling, the sampling velocity should be identical to the airflow velocity, so that there is neither dilution nor concentration of the aerosol within the sampling system.

Where the filter is not directly accessible for scanning, leaks can only be indirectly deduced by measuring the total amount of aerosol recovered downstream as a percentage of the amount introduced upstream. If the percent penetration is not within acceptable limits, the filter is deemed to be leaking.

Though it is easy to understand why the aerosol method has gained such widespread acceptance, it is not without serious deficiencies. Challenge aerosols are not, and do not behave like gases. They deposit on all available surfaces, which of course, includes the incident face of the filter under test, and the entire plenum chamber upstream of the filter. If the aerosol is hot, there is the additional problem of condensates. Besides the inevitably loading of the filter, this phenomenon makes estimation or maintenance of upstream challenge aerosol concentration very difficult.

To cut down on buildup of aerosol deposits on the filter, current trends are for diluting the challenge to as low as reasonably achievable levels (ALARA), taking into account the limit of detection (LOD) of the mass photometer. Good photometers are now available with a dynamic range of 1:10,000 or more. Hence, if upstream concentration is 100 μgrams/litre, downstream threshold concentration is 10 nanograms/litre. This has encouraged manufacturers and qualifiers of HEPAs and ULPAs to restrict upstream concentrations to 10 - 20 μgrams/litre for *probing for leaks* (integrity testing of filter in-situ), and selectively opting for full concentration of 100 μgrams/litre for *efficiency testing* at the factory. However, it must be emphasised that the pinhole behaviour of fibrous filters is sensitive to the aerosol flow rate, not concentration.

Alternatives to DOP: DOS (Di-octyl-sebacate); Shell's *Ondina* oil; White's *Kaydol*; BP Oiltech's *Enerpar*, a paraffin based oil; and Henkel's *Emery 3004*, a poly-alpha-olefein obtained by polymerising 1-decene saturated straight chain 20-carbon aliphatic hydrocarbon, methylene blue, corn oil, polystyrene-latex spheroids and tetra-ethylene glycol are some of the substances that are being experimented with, specially outside USA. Only Emery 3004 has received provisional approval from USFDA as an acceptable alternative to DOP.

Unfortunately all these alternatives are *oils* too. Apart from operational compatibility, toxicity, safety and other such considerations, the substance should lend itself to ready and convenient aerosolisation. The aerosol concentration is expressed in gravimetric terms (mg/m^3) but the photometer can only measure relative opacity, which is in photometric terms. Hence there should be a consistency in the correlation between the gravimetric and photometric concentration. In the case of DOP, for example, this correlation factor between gravimetric and photometric concentrations is 0.99, whereas for Emery 3004 it is 1.51. The correlation is influenced by physical characteristics like viscosity, change in viscosity with temperature, specific gravity, boiling point and refractive index.

The aerosoliser and photometer are generally calibrated for work with DOP; and require recalibration based on the correlation factor of the alternative challenge aerosol if the results are to be meaningful. The main changes are photometric recalibration, aerosolisation pressure and operating temperature.

The objective of aerosolisation is to produce a monodispersed challenge with count median diameter in the size range of interest to us (0.3μ) at a concentration that meets the test requirement. The number of particles N per litre of mean diameter D (μ) generated by aerosolising a substance of density ρ to a concentration of C (μg/litre) is given by the equation:

$$N = [6C/\pi\rho D^3] \times 10^6 \text{ per litre}$$

When thermal DOP is aerosolised, at a concentration of 100 μg/litre, we can expect a monondispersed population of 7.4×10^9 particles of 0.3μ/litre. This compares well with the typical contaminant density in the atmosphere (10^7 to 10^{11} per litre). If any alternative aerosol material is being used, the equation will help determine the size profile and density of droplets that will be produced.

Efficiency and Leak Tests with Particle Counters

In a photometer, the aerosol concentration is measured from the total light scattered by all the particles. That is, it does not discriminate particle sizes in

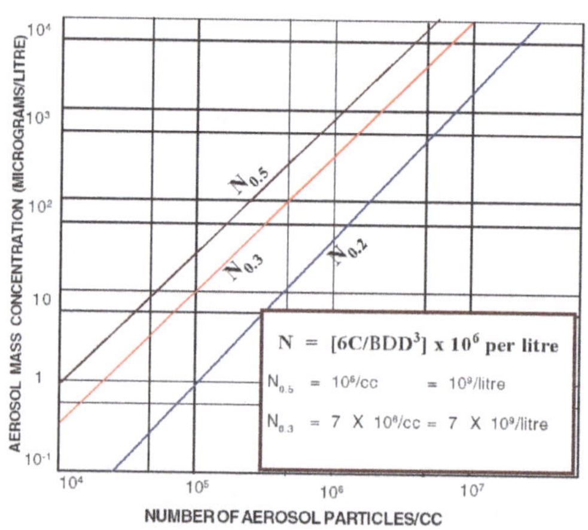

Fig. 6.5: DOP aerosol particles generator with a Laskin Nozzle

the aerosol and thus requires an aerosol of known size and size distribution. This device is the oldest of the filter test instrument. In its current designs, it is best suited for filter with efficiencies up to 99.999% and MPPS around 0.2 - 0.3µm. It is the preferred instrument for testing filters for pharmaceutical and nuclear applications.

An OPC measures the light scattered by individual particles rather than the entire aerosol. The strength of the scattered light is a measure of the particle size and the number of scattered light pulses a measure of the concentration. Thus the OPC is capable of measuring particle size distributions. As in all counting devices, its accuracy is dependent on the number of counts. Current designs are suitable for particles as small 0.1µm. The OPC is used widely for filters with efficiencies exceeding 99.99999%, limited only by the count statistics at the higher efficiencies.

In a CNC, the particles are introduced into a saturated vapor of a liquid. The particles act as nuclei to form a cloud of droplets due to heterogeneous nucleation. The droplets are then typically measured by optical scattering. The original designs of the CNC featured water and cooling by adiabatic expansion to effect the droplet formation. The current designs use alcohol and continuous flow with external cooling. Although the CNC counts individual droplets, individual particle size is lost since they only act as nuclei of the droplets counted. However, since even very small particles can act as a nucleus for droplet formation, the CNC is capable of counting particles as small as 0.05 µm. The CNC is currently increasingly used for microelectronics where the critical sizes are getting as small as 0.08µm and for filters of all efficiencies limited only by count statistics at the higher efficiencies.

Although all three instruments are commonly used for testing cleanroom filters, their results cannot be used inter changeably. Both the photometer and the CNC cannot discriminate particle size and hence require aerosol of known size or size distribution. Since the CNC can count particles of virtually any size, impurities in the system will also be counted leading to errors. The OPC requires dilution of the aerosol at higher concentrations to avoid thc counting of two coincident particles as one large particle. Further, the sensitivity of the OPC at smaller sizes is not as good as at larger sizes leading to count efficiency errors. For example, at particle sizes below 0.1µm, the CNC will count all particles, but particles counted by the OPC may be reduced by its count efficiency. Thus, the filter efficiency determined by the two instruments will be different. Also, efficiency determined using a photometer or a CNC is specific to the aerosol size or size distribution used. The OPC can determine the efficiency at any or all of the sizes within in its measurement range.

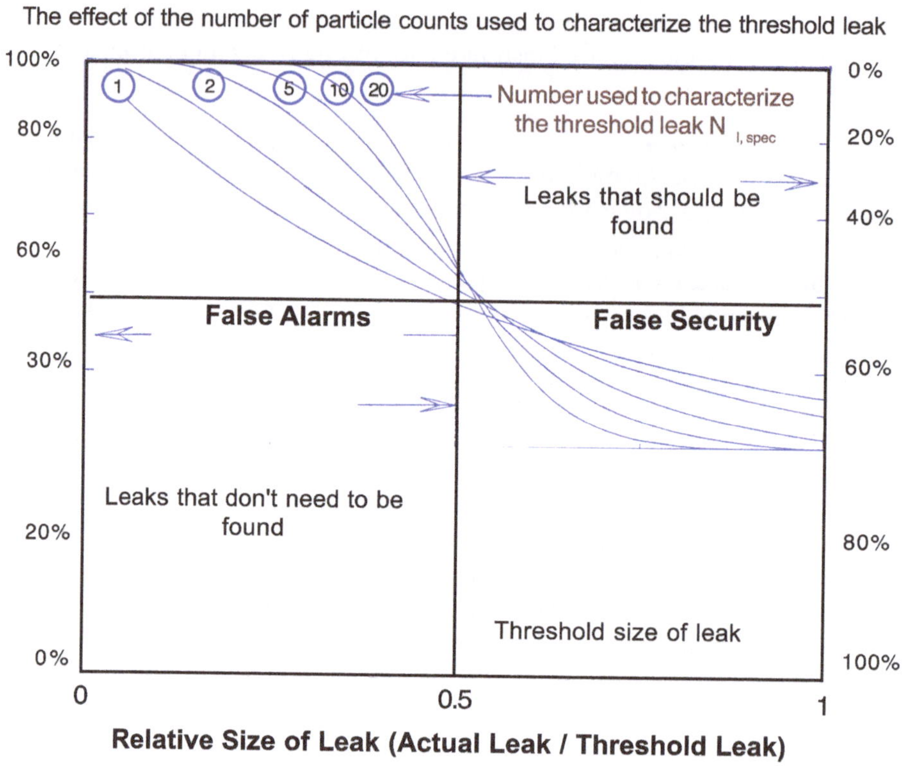

Fig. 6.6: Uncertainty in monitoring

Table 6.3: Recommended leak testing for different applications

Less than Class 100	Photometer scanning; Particle Counter not recommended. Application typically uses HEPA
Better than Class 100	Photometer or Particle Counter scanning. Photometer use depends on filter used
Microelectronics	Particle Counter scanning only. No oil aerosol. PSL preferred
Pharmaceutical	Photometer preferred practice. Particle Counter Scan with PSL if acceptable to user and FDA (in most cases)
Remote Filters	Total leak only, scanning not possible.

The probability of finding a leak is governed by the size of the probe, the responsiveness of the test instrument, and the rate of scanning. Smaller probes increase the ability to detect leaks since it samples smaller air volumes to dilute a leak thus amplifying any local leaks. Slower scanning speeds and more responsive instruments increase the ability to detect leaks. Smaller probes or slower scanning rates also increase the time needed to test a filter.

If a particle counting instrument, such as a CNC or an OPC, is used, the probability of detecting leaks is governed by the Poisson probability function.

Higher counts improve the ability to detect leaks and reduce false leaks. But increasing the required counts also extends the time required for testing, especially for higher efficiencies. The design of acceptable leak testing procedures is discussed in detail in IEST CC RP 034.1.

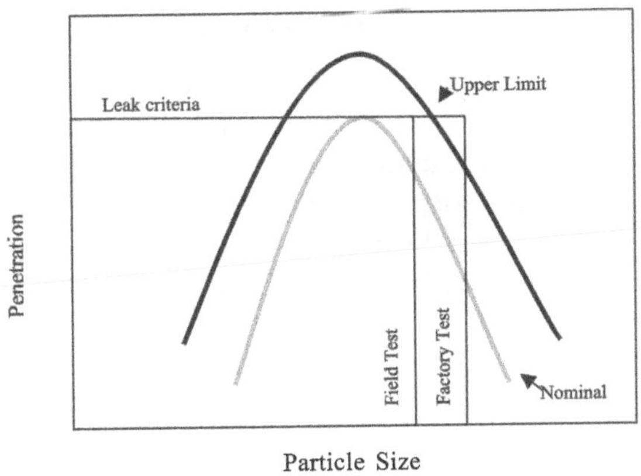

Figure 6.7: Problems with leak testing and particle size miss match

There are two common problems in testing cleanroom filters, specially using particle counters. When filter efficiencies are very high, the downstream concentrations can be very low. Long sample times are then required to obtain sufficient count statistics making routine filter testing impractical. For such high efficiency filters, it is current practice to accept the test results of filter media at the design velocity; test only a sample population of filters for efficiency; and leak test all filters. Thus, if the filter is verified to be leak free, then it is assumed that the efficiency is determined by the efficiency of the media.

The other problem is one of failure of a good filter during leak testing in the field. Most of the time this occurs due to a mismatch in the either test flows, or particle size or both and when setting leak test criteria close to the performance limits of the media. Leak is a local penetration and will measure the local variations in the media as shown qualitatively in Figure 6. Consider the case when the leak criteria is set at a larger particle size and just above the upper limit of the media If it is subsequently tested at a smaller particle size, the filter shows a leak. One may examine other combinations of mismatched particle sizes that lead to similar conflicting test results. The problem is exacerbated when different test flows are used. As discussed earlier, changing test flows changes penetration nearly exponentially greatly affecting test results. Thus, the growing trend in cleanrooms filter testing is to specify all filters and filter tests at its MPPS for the rated flow.

Qualifying Cleanrooms

Testing for continued compliance is governed by ISO 14644-2, and any other standard or guideline that the User may opt to abide by. Test methodologies and instrumentation are described in ISO 14644-3. Table 6.6 lists the parameters and their acceptance values, if applicable, as agreed between Buyer and Vendor.

Main air supply, make up air supply and reserve capacity

The purpose of these tests is to determine the main air supply volume introduced to the cleanroom, the volume of make up air delivered by the make up air handling system, and the reserve capacities of the air handling system, and the reserve capacities of the air handling systems to accommodate a loaded filter condition. The procedures are described in IES-RP-CC-006-84T and AMCA publication 203.

Air volume & uniformity

The test methodology and instrumentation to be used are described in the draft ISO 14644-3. The average air exchange rate is also determined during this procedure. IES-RP-CC-006.2 also describes the test, and includes air velocity and uniformity.

Airborne velocity & uniformity

ISO 14644-3 treats this as a separate exercise, whereas the earlier IEST document had clubbed it with airflow measurements.

Air velocity can be measured with a variety of anemometers. The windmill type probe is most reliable for wind speed measurements, and is not very accurate in the velocity ranges that apply in a cleanroom. Other mechanical types include the vane anemometer and the Pitot tube anemometer, the latter being more sensitive. The best results are attained with a thermo-anemometer. The probe must be held normal to airflow.

Air velocity mapping of the cleanroom is an important test exercise. But it is difficult to detect upward recirculatory flows, eddies and identify stagnant pockets in the room using only an anemometer.

Table 6.4 : Parameters for cleanroom & LAF Qualification

Parameter	References	Unidirectional	Turbulent	Mixed	Acceptance	
					Rooms	LF Devices
Main Air Supply Volume	ACMA 203				MA	N/A
Make up Air Supply Volume	ACMA 203				MA	N/A
Reserve Capacity of Main AHU	ACMA 203				MA	N/A
Air volume & uniformity	ISO 14644-3	1,2,3	1,2,3	1,2,3	5%	10%
Air velocity & uniformity	ISO 14644-3	1,2,3	O	O	5%	24 - 30 m/min
Airflow visualisation	ISO 14644-3				MA	MA
Airflow direction	ISO 14644-3				MA	MA
Installed Filter Leak	ISO 14644-3	1,2	1,2	1,2	0.01%	0.01%
Particle Count	ISO 14644-3	1,2,3	1,2,3	1,2,3	<UCL	MA
Ultrafines Count	ISO 14644-3				MA	MA
Macro-Particles Count	ISO 14644-3				MA	N/A
Microbial Count	MCA/WHO/M				MA	MA
Pressurisation	ISO 14644-3	1,2,3	1,2,3	1,2,3	MA	N/A
Parallelism[a]	ISO 14644-3	1,2	-	O (1,2 only)	14°	14°
Integrity/Containment Leak	ISO 14644-3	1,2	1,2	1,2	$< 10^{-3}$	0.01%
Induction/Back streaming	IES-RP-CC-002/6				$< 10^{-3}$	Nil
Recovery	ISO 14644-3	N/A	1,2	1,2	MA	N/A
Particle Fallout/Deposition	ISO 14644-3	1,2,3	1,2,3	1,2,3	MA	N/A
Lighting Level	IES-RP-CC-002/6	1,O (2,3)	1,O (2,3)	1,O (2,3)	MA	800 lumens/m^2
Electrostatic & Ion Generator	ISO 14644-3				MA	MA
Noise Level	IES-RP-CC-002/6	1,2	1,2	1,2	MA	< 67 dbA
Temperature uniformity	ISO 14644-3	1,2,3	1,2,3	1,2,3	(1 - 0.05 ^{o}C)	Rise < 5.6 ^{o}C
Moisture uniformity	ISO 14644-3	O	O	O	MA	N/A
Vibration	IES-RP-CC-002/6	O	O	O	MA	< 5μ rms at 10 - 200Hz

Airlow visualisation

To study how clean air entering the room is dispersed within the enclosed space before exiting, it is important to have some means of *visualising the air distribution pattern*. ISO 14644-3 and IES-RP-CC-006.2 both describe the methodology.

The test method should not compromise the integrity of the room by introducing elements that are difficult to eliminate after the test. *Smoke candles* were tried in the past, but their extreme corrosivity preclude their general use.

Mylar strips hung from the ceiling served the limited purpose of demonstrating turbulent effects caused by movement of personnel, apart from generally leaning in the direction of airflow.

Neutrally buoyant bubbles generated in a range of sizes as a cloud either at the air entry points or at a predetermined height from floor level. The manner in which these bubbles disperse can be photographed if necessary.

Cleanroom Foggers produce a high purity DI (deionized) water fog by condensing purified steam with liquid nitrogen by a unique, patented process. The water fog is neutrally buoyant, non-contaminating, highly visible and no residue particles are produced when the droplets evaporate. They are suitable for use in Class 1/10/100/ 1000/10000 cleanrooms for airflow and turbulence visualization, flow balancing, and contaminant transport studies around process tools. (*Other fog generators based on ultrasonic atomization or the dry-ice CO2 process create invisible residue particles when the droplets evaporate, making them unsuitable for use in Class 1/10/100 cleanrooms*).

Another emerging scientific way of anticipating and visualising airflow in cleanrooms is by solving for the physics of the problem using numerical methods known as *Computational Fluid Dynamics* (or CFD for short). In the mechanical ventilation design fraternity they are commonly known as Airflow Modeling techniques. These are mathematical modeling techniques used to solve for the physics of the complex fluid flow and heat transfer that occur in any real situation and are based on the Navker-Stokes equation.

Such test procedures shows up deficiencies in the air distribution system in a manner that no other method can approach, and helps designers fine tune the system for optimal performance.

Airflow direction

This is a new addition to the long list that has just appeared in the draft ISO 14644-3.

Installed Filter Leak

ISO 14644-3 and IES-RP-CC-006.2 are the reference documents.

This has been discussed at length in the earlier section on testing filters. Some points are worth repeating.

The probe should be held normal to the airflow, sampling should be isokinetic and the scan speed should not exceed 10 linear fpm. Where filter is accessible, distance of probe from filter face: 1" for LAF devices; 4" for terminally mounted filters and 6" for testing filter banks.

This critical *in situ* test is more often than not abused. Probing for leaks with a particular counter as against a photometer is itself a highly moot point. To compound the difficulty, use of atmospheric challenge makes it even more suspect an exercise, specially in an ultraclean environment where the ambient count, upstream or downstream is so low as place the readings beyond the LOD of the sensor.

Also as explained earlier, leaks show up best when air flow is reduced. If you recall, we had made the following important observations earlier on the section on air filters:

If there are pinhole leaks in the media, penetration will increase with decreasing airflow, relatively independent of particle size. This is because the constriction of airflow through a pinhole is a function of the air velocity whenever the constriction of air flow through the fibrous filter media. Therefore, at 20% or one-fifth of full test flow, a pinhole shows up as 5 times greater in proportion to total flow than it does at full flow. Also, at higher velocities particles impact upon the fibres of the filter element directly, whereas at lower velocities Brownian motion causes them to drift and wander. In the process they are more likely to find their way out of the leak.

Another reason is that as airflow reduces, the leakage of the challenge aerosol through the pinhole causes an increase in the concentration downstream. The "masking" effect caused by surrounding "clean" airstreams is less pronounced.

Particle counting, as mentioned earlier, is "an event" that obeys the Poisson Distribution in statistics where the mean of the population equals its variance. As the number of counts increase the distribution becomes increasingly "normal"; as the numbers decrease, it approaches the "binomial". Errors, both chance positives as well as chance negatives, can be very high indeed as cleanroom classifications approach ISO 4 and better.

Unfortunately, the new standards and test procedure guidelines somehow seem to have lost sight of this, and photometeric and aerosol photometric techniques seem to have lost out to particle counters as the method of choice for higher order cleanrooms.

IEST and other "Work Groups" are still actively wrestling with this contentious issue, and their documents may yet offer some relief, if not immediately, at some future date.

Airborne Particle Count

Air cleanliness is an expression of the particle density in the environment. If we sample a unit volume, the contaminant count gives us the contaminant density. Which is exactly what is sought to be achieved by *airborne particle counters*.

Rather than dwelling on the mechanical details of a particle counter, we focus on the special problems with the exercise. While all imaginable size objects can appear in the air, the mean (Geometric Mean Diameter) of the distribution is typically around 0.3μ. Since visible light lies in the spectrum of 0.4μ to 0.7μ light is not absorbed by the particle sought to be counted, since the path length required for absorption is inadequate; instead scatter effect predominates, with the index of refraction of the particle assuming prominence, and energy of scatter is a function of the entire particle, no longer a surface phenomenon. The particle size being of the order of the incident wavelength, the behaviour is like an antenna; and if the size is equal to or a multiple of the

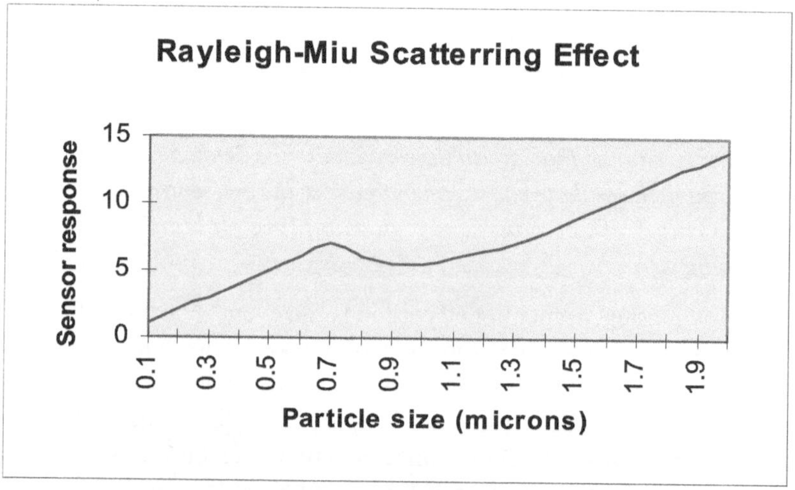

Fig. 6.8: "Blind Band" around 1μ with most OPCs

wavelength, the effect is like a tuned antenna. Under normal circumstances, conductive materials absorb light well; but their higher refractive indices prevent light from entering altogether when the size lies in this region. In fact, at the range 0.4μ to 0.7μ the limit of interaction between particle and illumination is reached, independent of signal to noise ratio. At sizes below the visible limit, the change in the intensity of scatter is several orders of magnitude for every order of change in particle size, rendering them invisible to the sensor.

As mentioned in Chapter 2, particles in air appear in every conceivable shape, not all of which are "regular" spheres. How do we characterise an irregular object? A fibre may be 30μ in length, and only 0.7μ in diameter. Are we looking at a 30μ object or at a 0.7μ object? Scientists have overcome this problem by introducing a concept called *equivalent* diameter to characterise irregular shapes. The equivalent diameter is the diameter of a reference sphere having known properties and producing the same response in the sensing instrument as the particle being measured. While it is mathematically convenient, we must not lose sight of this approximation.

We have mentioned earlier that in any normal air sample, though the bigger particles are fewer than the smaller particles, they represent a larger proportion of the total weight. Thus the "equivalent" diameter of the median particle of the population would be influenced by whether the distribution is arranged mass-wise or size-wise. The former is the Mass Median Diameter; the latter the Count Median Diameter. In particle counting, we normally refer to the latter only.

Since the typical atmospheric contaminant density is in billions and the air cleanliness sought to be achieved in the controlled environment often permits only single digits, the dynamic range of the particle counter must be very high indeed if the Limit of Detection (LOD) and threshold sensitivity in terms of both particle size and numbers is to be acceptable for meaningful testing in the cleanroom.

Rayleigh-Miu scattering curves confirm the presence of a "blind" band in the range 0.7μ to 1.3μ where the curve has a "kink" and the detected pulse amplitude does not have a unique correspondence in terms of particle size. Thus the instrument is unable to distinguish among, say 0.65μ, 0.9μ and 1.2μ! Instrument manufacturers have circumvented this problem with built-in context-sensitive correction coefficients.

A pump within the counter draws in the air sample. This pump, like any other pump, performs well when operated within its intended range, and is less reliable outside it. Counters designed to draw 1 cfm have a larger pump than one designed to sample 0.1 or 0.01 cfm. In the latter two cases, the count is internally multiplied to give the final reading on the panel. Such miniature pumps have no difficulty aspirating submicronic particles; but they lack the strength to draw larger particles. As a result, the count of 0.3μ and 0.5μ particles in the sample may be reasonably accurate, but the value indicated for 5μ particles could be far from the actual.

Sampled air is routed through the probe and connected tubing to the sample cell before being exhausted. As everywhere else, suspended particles in the sample may sediment out, and other forces at play will cause further depositions, the convolutions in the sample path further accelerating the process. As a consequence, the number of particles counted may not be equal to the number of particles that were sampled. Sudden jerky movements with the probe or agitation of the tubing may produce artifacts caused by the dislodgment and re-entrainment of settled particles.

This deficiency is pronounced when sampling oil-laden air, like DOP aerosol for example, which can smear the entire sample path with a fine film of oil and even damage the optics (notwithstanding the protective sheath of purge air designed to preclude clouding of the sample cell). It would therefore be prudent to avoid using particle counters for testing with artificial challenge aerosols.

An important point to bear in mind is that the particle counter set to count a particular size, say 1μ and above, it will detect all particles of that size and larger. If challenged with an aerosol with that size as the *count median value*, it will detect only 50% of the population whose size is equal to or exceeds 1μ, since the remaining 50% would lie in the normal distribution below the *count median* threshold. This is known in particle counting parlance as the *50% count.*

A particle counter is calibrated using a challenge of nebulised monodispersed polystyrene latex spheres. In the past this facility was available only with instrument manufacturers, but models recently introduced feature an integral nebuliser. Since these are delicate instruments liable to go out of calibration often, periodic recalibration is good practice. In the absence of a built-in nebuliser, secondary calibration is done using another particle counter (which hopefully has been calibrated) as a reference instrument.

The sampling probe may be cylindrical or rectangular, though, as mentioned earlier, the current preference is toward the latter, for better scanning of filter edges and boundaries. Scanning distance, speed and general procedure is identical with that explained for photometers. Isokinetic sampling is particularly important if the results obtained are not to be undervalued or exaggerated. But isokinetic sampling is more easily said than done. The procedure for ascertaining the number of sample locations and number of samples per location are detailed in ISO 14644.

Continuous/On-line Particle Counting

Manufacturers of airborne particle counters have cause to cheer the new guidelines that are advocating installation of on-line monitoring of particle counts. I shall, too, on the day I am convinced that the system works reliably, repeatedly and reproducibly. Today if I pull a soft cloth through the probe tubing I find it gets soiled; if I tap the tube the reading jerks with artifacts. Just as a depth filter tends to trap airborne particles through sedimentation, impaction and other methods described in earlier sections, the probe tubing too behaves like a filter. All suspended particles may not have been "pulled in" (specially the "heavy" particles); all particles entering the probe may not make the distance to the sensing cell; and the reading understated. In on-line multi-point remote sampling probes, 30 feet of tubing, manifolds and centralised monitoring, this "deficiency" is likely to leave the User with data which in reality may be incomplete, but which he assumes is reliable. The miss of counts, specially of the larger particles, the likely carriers of viable organisms is a major drawback. Remember that a bacteria needs a carrier that is generally 10 times its own size. If the bacterial size range is, say, 0.3μ to 3μ, the carrier sizes we are looking at lies in the range 3μ to 30μ.

Ultrafines Count

This has been added in the new ISO 14644-3 document, which also describes the methodology; but how reliable the readings will be is another proposition altogether. Considering that the new wafer fab facilities are being commissioned for line widths in the range of 0.13μ, and the ones in the pipeline are aspiring for 0.08μ ultrafines measurements will prove increasingly critical over the coming years.

Macro-Particles Count

This too has been added in the new ISO 14644-3 document. But I fear that the results using regular airborne particle counters may need to be correlated with other measurement procedures. Perhaps back to the optical microscope techniques.

Pressurisation

The purpose of this test is to verify the capability of the cleanroom system to maintain the specified pressure gradients between the clean areas and their surroundings when doors are closed as well as when they are open. Acceptance criteria are indicated in some guidance documents; others leave it to the Buyer and Vendor to mutually agree upon. The range varies from 2.5 pascals (0.25 mm or 0.01" wc) to 15 pascals (1.5 mm or 0.06" wc) between adjacent areas.

Parallelism

The purpose of this test is to verify the parallelism of airflow throughout the work zone, and to check whether the cleanroom is capable of limiting the dispersion of internally generated contamination. Methodologies are described in ISO 14644-3 and IES-RP-CC-006.2. The work zone is generally divided into grids of 10' x 10' and the "entrance" plane and "exit" plane are defined, separated by at least 3'. The deviation or offset should normally lie within 14°.

Enclosure Integrity/Containment Leak

This test is performed to determine if there is intrusion or ingress of unfiltered or less clean air from surrounding areas into the clean work space: from outside the cleanroom enclosure through seams, joints and doorways. The ingress should, of course, be demonstrated to be nil. Refer IES-RP-CC-006.2 and ISO 14644-3.

Induction/Back streaming

Similar to the integrity test, but directed more toward LAF work stations: ingress of unfiltered or less clean air from outside the LAF work station into the work space through side panels and other joints. Refer IES-RP-CC-002.

Recovery test

This test is to determine whether the cleanroom or clean zone is capable of returning to its specified cleanliness class within a finite, predictable time after being exposed briefly to an artificially induced excursion beyond prescribed limits. Refer IES-RP-CC-006.2 and ISO 14644-3.

Particle Fallout/Deposition

This is one of the most useful tests, least practised. Regardless of the background count and airflow distribution, contamination is caused by fallout of contaminant on to the product, and it is often considered that the fallout rates and patterns are as crucial as airborne suspended counts. This test is performed to also measure levels of large particles, which are not effectively counted by airborne particle counters. Particle fallout measurements are obtained by allowing a small test surface (witness plate) to collect natural particles (no artificial challenge) which settle out naturally in the cleanroom environment. The particles on the witness plate are counted with a microscope, manual or automatic, and the particle settling rate is determined:

$$\frac{\text{Average particles}}{\text{cm}^2} = \frac{\text{Total particles on witness plate}}{\text{Witness plate area in cm}^2}$$

Witness plates should be cleaned before they are exposed. At least three witness plates should be used as controls, which are not exposed. The test plates should be exposed for four hours, or as long as is necessary to obtain a statistically valid sample, in as many critical locations as required, with a minimum of three witness plates per test location.

$$\text{Sedimentation rate} = \frac{\text{After Exposure Test count} - \text{Control Plate Count}}{\text{Area of witness plate in cm}^2}$$

This test complements the other test measurements carried out to provide a comprehensive status of environment particle levels for an as-built, at-rest, or operating facility. The choice of witness plate material should match the instrument intended to be used for surface particle detection. Refer IES-RP-CC-006.2 and ISO 14644-3.

Lighting Level

This test determines whether the lighting levels and lighting uniformity within the room are being met. Acceptance requires shadowless uniform lighting at intensity levels of 75 to 100 foot candles or 800 - 1076 lux (lumens/m^2). Refer IES-RP-CC-006.2 and ISO 14644-3.

Electrostatic & Ion Generator

This has been just introduced in ISO 14644-3; earlier references are given below.

ANSI EOS/ESD STM3.1 - 2000: Ionisation. This standard covers test methods and procedures for evaluating and selecting air ionisation equipment and systems. The document establishes measurement techniques to determine ion balance and charge neutralisation time for ionisers.

ESD ADV3.2 - 1995: Selection and Acceptance of Air Ionisers. This document provides end users with guidelines for selecting air ionisation systems. It reviews four types of air ionisers and discusses applications, test method references, and general design, performance and safety requirements.

Noise Level

The purpose of this test is to measure the airborne sound pressure levels produced by the basic cleanroom mechanical and electrical systems within the room and in adjacent external occupied areas and verify that performance meets the acceptance criteria, which is normally < 67 dB on A scale with a background ambient noise level < 55dB A. Refer IES-RP-CC-002 and ISO 14644-3.

Temperature and Moisture uniformity

ISO 14644-3 treats these as separate tests; but IES-RP-CC-006.2 had clubbed them together. The purpose is to determine and demonstrate the capability of the cleanroom air handling system to maintain air temperature and moisture (expressed as relative humidity or dew point) levels within the control limits and over the time period specified. Both documents offer detailed methodologies to be followed.

Vibration

The purpose is to determine vibration levels on the cleanroom structure and components. Refer IES-RP-CC-006/024 and ISO 14644-3. For LAF work stations refer IES-RP-CC-002, which recommends < 5μ rms at 10 - 200Hz.

Microbial Count

ISO 14698 is a set of three standards being developed to assist the User with drawing up comprehensive systems and procedures for bioaerosol monitoring and control. The standard does not prescribe specifics, but suggests elaborate schemes that help set target, alarm and action levels that must be mutually agreed between Buyer and Vendor. However, Orange Guide 2002, WHO 2002 and Schedule M have clearly prescribed acceptance levels.

Methods for determination of *airborne microorganisms* can be divided into four groups, according to the principle used: *Sedimentation*, *Impaction*, *Filtration* and *Impingement*. Since airborne microorganisms often form aggregates with each other or with suspended particles, counting them individually is not always possible. If we collect airborne microbes on an agar nutrient plate, each aggregate can grow to give one *colony*. Thus the resulting colonies give us the number of aggregates or *colony forming units* (CFU) in the air sample.

The *sedimentation* method is simple and inexpensive. Petri dishes, containing agar nutrient medium, are opened in the area to be tested and exposed for a predetermined interval. They are then closed and incubated. The sedimented aggregates form colonies, and these are simply counted.

One disadvantage is that the count so obtained cannot be related to any specific air volume. The fallout rate being probabilistic, the results are not strictly repeatable. Since large agglomerates fall more rapidly than individual microbes, the count is more representative of the former, rather than the total airborne microbial density. Besides, there is little consensus of opinion among experts on exposure times and corresponding CFU counts that may be deemed acceptable. Notwithstanding all these drawbacks, this is the method that most closely simulates the probability of fallout contamination of the product, since the same effects that influence the sedimentation rate on the test plate apply to the product as well.

Impaction type samplers force air onto a moist surface of an agar plate, so that particles and airborne microbes stick to the surface. The *Slit Sampler* (so named because it draws air through a slit located overhead), has a rotating agar plate to help distribute the microorganisms over the entire plate. The *Agar Drum Sampler*, where agar is spun on to a drum under sterile conditions uses a ventilator with vertical blades to draw the air in past the agar drum and centrifuge the microorganisms on to the agar surface. The *Reuter Centrifugal Air Sampler*, slightly larger than a flashlight, is an example, and is among the most popular models. The *Anderson Sampler* even separates the particles collected according to their size. It contains six agar plates, one in each stage, and the air is drawn through a series of sieve plates, which have smaller and smaller hole sizes (1.18 mm to 0.25 mm). Since the air velocity depends on the cross-section of flow, it is accelerated at each stage. The larger particles ($>8\mu$) are collected in the upper most stage and the submicronic in the lowest. The deficiency common to impaction and centrifugal type samplers is the rapid drying out of the agar surface, low retentivity leading to loss of viability and the shear forces that cause breakdown of agglomerates resulting in misleading higher counts on the one hand and damage to cells on the other.

Filtration air samplers cause air to pass through a series of filter membranes of decreasing porosity, which are then placed directly on a nutrient plate containing the culturing medium of choice. The filter dissolves on the moist surface, so that the microorganisms are in direct contact with the nutrients. The plates are incubated and the colonies counted. Drying out of the membrane often causes loss of viability and retention, though when gelatin is used in place of cellulose, there is a marked improvement in retention. Another disadvantage lies in the decreasing sample airflow with increased filter loading. Shear forces cause de-agglomeration and sometimes damage sensitive cells.

The impinger air sampler draws test air directly into the collecting medium with the aid of a vacuum source. The airflow rate is regulated. Since the microbes are drawn into the collecting medium and intimately mixed deep within, the retention is high and there is no danger of loss of viability due to drying out of the agar surface. Though there is no shear force or acceleration, if air velocity is not maintained within threshold limit, there is danger of de-agglomeration. The pre-sampling effort is easy; post-sampling exercise may, however, require extended work and elaborate laboratory set up.

In all designs of air samplers it is necessary to keep the air sampling time short for optimum results. Except in the sedimentation method, which is non-volumetric, air sampling must be isokinetic.

Multi-location intermittent or continuous on-line sampling, both sequential as well as simultaneous, has become technically feasible for airborne microbes.

Contact surface sampling uses Replicate Organisms Detection and Counting (RODAC) dishes, usually 55 mm diameter, into which 15.5 to 16 ml of agar medium is poured. The agar meniscus gives the dish a convex shape, facilitating its roll over surface to be sampled. Microbes adhere to the agar, and the dish is then incubated. Additives may be added to the agar medium to neutralise residual disinfectants that may otherwise inhibit microbial growth.

Agar contact strips may also be used for surface sampling. Strips are removed from their container and applied to the surface. Microbes adhere to the strip, which is then incubated.

Swabbing is commonly used to sample uneven surfaces. A cotton bud swab is first rubbed on the surface being sampled and then rubbed over an agar plate, which is then incubated. For improved efficiency and reproducibility the swab is generally dampened with sterile saline. Shaking the swab in a container with agar, or dropping the swab inside the agar are also techniques employed. Aliquots are prepared, filtered and incubated.

Alternative detection techniques: A number of alternative methods are being designed for detecting and enumerating microbes.

Epifluorescence Microscopy is a rapid method for enumerating bacteria, and the counts so obtained are of several orders of magnitude greater than those obtained by culture methods. These counts are composites of viable and culturable, viable and non-culturable, anaerobic and nonviable cells. This method, however, cannot identify the species.

On the other hand, Scanning Electron Microscopy not only determines the morphological diversity in the biofilm, but also estimates the numbers and

Table 6.5: Biological Monitoring Summary

* **Three stages of microbial level measurement**
    1. Taking a representative sample
    2. Examination
    3. Interpretation

* **Estimating the bioburden/profiling of people**
    1. Finger dabs
    2. Glove prints
    3. Swabs from gown and exposed parts of body

* **Estimating aerial bioburden**
    1. *Active sampling*

a. Slit-to-Agar	(Cassella/Reynier)
b. Sieve samplers	(Anderson)
c. Centrifugal	(Reuters)
d. Liquid samplers	(Sartorius Impingement Air Sampler)
e. Filtration	

    2. *Passive sampling*

a. Sedimentation	(Petri dish/ settle plate)
b. Simulated fills	(Broth runs)

* **Estimating surface bioburden**

a. Swab	
b. Agar contact	(RODAC plate)
c. Agar overlay	

* **Sampling location**

* **Rapid methods**
    a. Epifluorescence
    b. Bioluminescence
    c. Total Organic Carbon

distributions of attached or free bacteria, and the overall extent of the surface population. Organic carbon serves as a colonisation stratum for bacteria, which in turn are actively involved in recycling the organic carbon. Since there is a direct correlation, Total Organic Carbon (TOC) measurements can help estimate the bacterial number.

Table 6.6: Environment Monitoring: Study of Alternate Methods

Method	Advantages	Disadvantages
Slit-to-Agar	Very efficient Samples large volume Plate directly incubated	Bulky, intrusive Adjustment critical May dry out
Sieve sampler	Efficient Intermediate volumes Single-stage, non-intrusive Plate directly incubated of particles	Single stage not commercially available. Current one on market expels large numbers
Centrifugal	Portable Manipulatable Plate directly incubated	Sample volume not known. Strips available from only one supplier. Samples small volume
Liquid sampler	Very efficient Total number of bacteria in sample can be determined	Clumsy, fragile, needs plating out
Filtration		
Membrane	Efficient Samples large volumes	Dries and kills bacteria Needs plating separately
Gelatine	Efficient Samples large volumes May give total number of bacteria per unit volume	Only availble from one supplier. Needs plating step
Settle plates	Cheap, easy to use, one step	Sampling volume not known, but not large. May dry out
Broth runs	Predicts actual contamination rate. Good as a validation exercise	Expensive in terms of production time. Difficult to evaluate

Microorganisms may also be evaluated by assays developed to measure specific components that are found in their cells. Some components like protein and carbohydrates are found in all living cells; but some are associated uniquely with specific groups (for example, lipopolysaccharide in gram negative bacteria). Although the quantities of these components vary within microbial cells, they are often used as a measure of microbial biomass.

Table 6.7: Surface Monitoring - Study of Alternate Methods

Method	Advantages	Disadvantages
Surface swab	Cheap Qualitative Easy with practice	Relies on frictional transfer. Use of preservative antagonizes. Poor efficiency
Contact	Cheap Semi-quantitative Easy with practice	Relies on adhesion Efficiency 20% - 70% Leaves nutrient film behind
Agar overlay	Very efficient Quantitative	Clumsy Need supply of inert strips

Table 6.8

Microorganism type	Culture medium	Incubation	
		^{0}C	hrs
Acid-tolerant bacteria	Orange serum	32	48
Colony count	Standard Nutrient agar Trypticase Soy agar Sabouraud Dextrose agar	32 32 RT	48 48 96
Colony count & hemolytic effect of Staphylococci & Streptococci	Sheep Blood agar DST Blood agar	37 37	48 48
Pediococci & Lactobacilli	NBB agar VLB-S-7 agar	32 32	48 48
Yeasts & Moulds	Sabouraud Dextrose agar Wort agar	RT 32	96 48

Concluding remarks

Irrespective of the type of testing, the qualification programme must clearly lay down parametric limits signifying acceptable values, and multi-tiered limits (*target, routine notification*, *alert* or *alarm* levels) when deviations occur, so that concerned personnel may initiate appropriate remedial action before things get out of hand.

A test report should ideally be in the form of a historical record of parametric values, so that trends may be easily discerned.

Today's documentation demands, however, require far more.

Model Cleanroom Testing Specifications issued by ***National Environmental Balancing Bureau***, and *Validation of Controlled Environment in a Parenteral Facility* reproduced in the following pages are representative examples, though their document, nomenclature and references are still to the pre-ISO era.

National Environmental Balancing Bureau

8575 Grovemont Circle
Gaithersburg, Maryland 20877

MODEL CLEANROOM TESTING SPECIFICATIONS

The following specification for *Cleanroom Certification and Acceptance Procedures* may be incorporated into the contract documents by the specifying authority. NEBB *Qualified Cleanroom Performance Testing (CPT) Supervisors* are fully cognizant of the obligations contained in the following specification and in the NEBB *Procedural Standards for Certified Testing of Cleanrooms,* Second Edition—1996. They have received extensive education in cleanroom performance testing and have successfully passed written and practical examinations to comply with certification requirements. They also annually attend specified national educational seminars to update and add to their expertise.

The NEBB *Certified Cleanroom Performance Testing (CPT) Firm* must employ at least one qualified NEBB CPT Supervisor and meet all other written requirements by NEBB to maintain certification through biennial recertification.

CLEANROOM CERTIFICATION AND ACCEPTANCE PROCEDURES

PART I—GENERAL

1.1 Work Included *[Edit this specification to eliminate tests not required. Place tests in the desired sequence of performance]*

A. This section provides the services required by the NEBB Certified Cleanroom Performance Testing (CPT) Firm hereinafter referred to as the *NEBB CPT Firm,* to measure and record the cleanroom conditions and resolve all nonconforming areas prior to attesting that the cleanroom is complete and ready for Owner's testing and occupancy.

B. At completion of the certification period, the Owner may engage the services of an independent quality assurance testing and certifying agency to perform random spot checks of all data collected during the NEBB CPT Firm's certifying period. This quality assurance agency, if used, will act only on behalf of the Owner to ensure that certification measurements and data are within industry tolerances and will verify that space conditions and system operations have not changed.

C. The NEBB CPT Firm shall perform the following (checked off) tests described below.

1. Airflow Velocity and Uniformity Tests
2. HEPA Filter Installation Leak Tests.
3. Room Particle Count Tests.
4. Enclosure Pressurization Tests.
5. Temperature and Humidity Uniformity Tests.
6. Sound and Vibration Tests.
7. Light Level and Uniformity Tests
8. Recovery Tests.
9. Conductivity Tests.
10. Particle Fallout Count Tests.
11. Electrostatic Tests.

D. NEW CONSTRUCTION (Optional): the NEBB CPT Supervisor shall visit the job site a minimum of once every [_____] weeks during the period that construction work is being performed on the *finished* cleanroom to review and make inspections of the cleanroom HVAC systems. The cost of the time and associated expense for these visits shall be included in the proposal.

E. HEPA/ULPA Filter Repair and Replacement: If defective ceiling filters are identified during the course of the certification testing, the NEBB CPT Firm shall immediately notify the Owner, and repair or replacement shall be performed at the direction of the owner and at mutually agreed fees or costs.

1.2 Related Sections

A. This section shall be used in conjunction with the following other specifications and related Contract Documents to establish the total requirements for the referenced cleanroom testing and certification.

1. Section _____
2. Section _____
3. Section _____
4. Division 1—General Requirements
5. Cleanroom Drawings and specifications.

CAUTION ! Use of this section without including all of the previously listed items will result in omission of basic requirements.

B. In the event of conflict regarding requirements for the referenced cleanroom testing and certification between this section and any other section, the provisions of this section shall govern.

1.3 References

A. Federal Standard 209E, *Airborne Particulate Cleanliness Class for Cleanrooms and Clean Zones:*

B. IES-RP-CC-006.2-1993, *Testing Cleanrooms* and IES-RP-CC-001.3-1993, *HEPA and ULPA Filters*:

C. NEBB *Procedural Standards for Certified Testing of Cleanrooms, Second Edition—1996.*

1.4 System Description

A. Definitions

B. Class of clean areas shall be as listed below:

____

____

____

1.5 Warranty

A. The service to be furnished by the NEBB CPT Firm *should be* considered complete and accepted when the Cleanroom Certification Test Report has been approved by the Owner.

1.6 Quality Assurance

A. All cleanroom air systems should be tested and certified by a nationally certified firm specializing in cleanroom certification. The NEBB CPT Firm shall review the work of construction trades required to complete construction of the cleanrooms in accordance with the Construction Documents (see 1.01-D).

B. NEBB CPT Firms shall have been in business a minimum of [_____] years specializing in cleanroom testing and certifying work. A list shall be available upon request, of projects similar in size, complexity, and cleanliness classification similar to this project that the firm has completed. Include the project name, description of mechanical systems, range of services provided, and the name and phone number of the design consultant and the owner who were responsible for final acceptance of the service.

1.7 Submittals

A. Submittals shall be provided in accordance with Section [_____]—Submittals, and the requirements of this section.

B. The following are required with the proposal:

6. [_____] copies of the completed Cleanroom Certification Report shall be submitted for the Owner's review and acceptance.

1.8 Job Conditions

A. Certification shall not proceed until all other work on the cleanroom has been completed and the commencement of certification work has been approved.

B. Condition of Cleanrooms Prior to Testing:

   1. The HVAC system installation for the cleanroom, including all of the exhaust systems and makeup air systems associated with the cleanroom operation, should have been completed, including all air and hydronic testing, adjusting, and balancing work, and a TAB report submitted.
   2. All floor tiles shall be in place, and all wall and ceiling penetrations sealed to airflow.

PART 2—PRODUCTS *[Edit to eliminate items not required]*

2.1 Materials

A. The NEBB CPT Firm shall supply all [materials], tools, [equipment], and instrumentation required to perform the cleanroom system testing and certification as described in this section. Cleanroom garments *not* included.

B. Once the cleanroom has been installed (select one of the following): only [a polystyrene latex (PSL) aerosol], [Di-Ethyl-Hexyl-Sebecate (DEHS) aerosol (C26H5004)], [DOP aerosol], [_______________] shall be used for challenge of [HEPA] [ULPA] filters.

2.2 Instrumentation

A. Only approved state-of-the-art test equipment and instrumentation shall be used in the certification test procedures as described in Chapter 14—*Equipment and Instrumentation* of the NEBB *Procedural Standards for Certified Testing of Cleanrooms, Second Edition—1996.*

B. The approved test instrumentation shall be used as described in the certification test procedures found in the NEBB *Procedural Standards for Certified Testing of Cleanrooms, Second Edition—1996.*

PART 3—EXECUTION

3.1 Preparation

A. The NEBB CPT Firm shall supervise and conduct all tests in the presence of the Owner's representative.

B. The as-built cleanroom certification tests shall be performed after the HVAC TAB work has been completed and the Owner's representative is satisfied that the installation is ready for certification testing. Final clean down [and commissioning procedures] also shall be completed.

C. All cleanroom recirculation fans, makeup air fans, process fume exhaust systems, and automatic control loops shall be in operation during tests. All mechanical systems and all fans related to cleanroom systems shall be verified to be operating as specified and delivering design airflow.

D. Tests described below are not identified necessarily in their proper sequence. The sequence of test procedures shall be as stated in the Proposal.

3.2 Field Testing and Certifying Procedures

A. Airflow Velocity and Uniformity Tests
Follow the cleanroom certification test procedures found in Chapter 5—*Airflow Test Procedures* of the NEBB *Procedural Standards for Certified Testing of Cleanrooms, Second Edition—1996.*

B. HEPA Filter Installation Leak Tests.
Follow the cleanroom certification test procedures found in Chapter 6—*HEPA Filter Installation Leak Testing* of the NEBB *Procedural Standards for Certified Testing of Cleanrooms, Second Edition—1996.*

C. Room Particle Count Tests
Follow the cleanroom certification test procedures found in Chapter 7—*Room Cleanliness Classification Testing* of the NEBB *Procedural Standards for Certified Testing of Cleanrooms, Second Edition—1996.*

D. Enclosure Pressurization Tests

Follow the cleanroom certification test procedures found in Chapter 8—*Enclosure Pressurization and Integrity Testing* of the NEBB *Procedural Standards for Certified Testing of Cleanrooms, Second Edition—1996.*

E. Temperature and Humidity Uniformity Tests

Follow the cleanroom certification test procedures found in Chapter 10—*Temperature and Humidity Testing* of the NEBB *Procedural Standards for Certified Testing of Cleanrooms, Second Edition—1996.*

F. Sound and Vibration Tests

Follow the cleanroom certification test procedures found in Chapter 9—*Sound and Vibration Testing* of the NEBB *Procedural Standards for Certified Testing of Cleanrooms, Second Edition—1996.*

G. Light Level and Uniformity Tests

Follow the cleanroom certification test procedures found in Chapter 11—*Lighting Level and Uniformity Testing* of the NEBB *Procedural Standards for Certified Testing of Cleanrooms, Second Edition—1996.*

H. Recovery Tests

Follow the cleanroom certification test procedures found in Section 12.1—*Recovery Test* of Chapter 12 of the NEBB *Procedural Standards for Certified Testing of Cleanrooms, Second Edition—1996.*

I. Conductivity Test

Follow the cleanroom certification test procedures found in Section 12.3—*Conductivity Tests* of Chapter 12 of the NEBB *Procedural Standards for Certified Testing of Cleanrooms, Second Edition—1996.*

J. Particle Fallout Count Tests

Follow the cleanroom certification test procedures found in Section 12.2—*Particle Fallout*

Count Test of Chapter 12 of the NEBB *Procedural Standards for Certified Testing of Cleanrooms, Second Edition—1996.*

K. Electrostatic Tests

Follow the cleanroom certification test procedures found in Section 12.4—*Electrostatic Tests* of Chapter 12 of the NEBB *Procedural Standards for Certified Testing of Cleanrooms, Second Edition—1996.*

3.3 Acceptance Criteria

A. Verification Procedures

1. If specified, the NEBB CPT Firm shall demonstrate to the Owner's representative, the test instrumentation to be used and the certification performance test procedures to be followed.
2. At the completion of all certification performance tests, the NEBB CPT Supervisor shall review all certification test data with the Owner's representatives and establish the base operating condition of cleanrooms and clean spaces.

B. Documentation

1. The NEBB CPT Supervisor shall review the certification test report data for compliance after each test, and then sign/ stamp the final reports for submittal to the Owner.
2. The NEBB CPT Firm shall deliver [_____] complete sets of all certification [data] [logs] in bound form to the Owner.

Validation of Controlled Environment in a Parenteral Facility

Sample Standard Operating Procedure

Purpose and Scope

To detail the Environmental Quality Assurance Department (EQA) as it relates to the validation of controlled environments defined as:

Class 100 ... Sterile

Class 10,000... Clean

Class 100,000 ... Ancillary

This procedure will apply to all newly constructed, upgraded or existing controlled environments

Responsibilities

Responsibilities are clearly defined below. However, EQA will provide the necessary assistance and support to local personnel to assure that the prevalidation and validation requirements are fulfilled.

A. EQA will be responsible for

1. Approving the draft blueprints and design specifications for new or upgraded controlledenvironments based on the requirements specified in the Worldwide Standard for Sterile Manufacturing and Sterility Testing.
2. Approving the as-built blueprints and design specifications of existing controlled environments based on the minimum design criteria specified
3. Reviewing and filling the prevalidation documentation as specified
4. Conducting a review of the physical characteristics of the controlled environments, if required
5. Providing on-site support, if required by local personnel

B. Local personnel will be responsible for:

1. Notifying EQA in writing during the design phase of new or upgraded controlled environments
2. For new or upgraded controlled environments, submitting to EQA for approval draft blueprints and design specifications

3. For existing controlled environments submitting to EQA as-built blueprints and design specifications
4. Submitting prevalidation documentation to EQA before the validation begins for both new orupgraded controlled environments and for existing controlled environments, unless otherwise noted. The prevalidation documentation must include the following:
   a. EQA approved blueprints and reference flow diagrams for new or upgraded controlled environments
   b. A system description and design specifications of the controlled environments
5. Having the following documentation on file at the local facility:
   a. A list of operating manuals for the components of the controlled environments
   b. A statement verifying that for new or upgraded controlled environments, a system blow down, balancing and DOP certification was performed for the HVAC system in accordance with local Standard Operating Procedure requirements. For laminar flow modules, a statement verifying that there was an initial blow down and DOP certification in accordance with local Standard Operating Procedure requirements.
   c. A list of all instruments and recording devices installed in the controlled environments and HVAC system, and a statement verifying that each was calibrated to manufacturers' specifications in accordance with local Standard Operating Procedure requirements.
6. Qualification test results for newly constructed and upgraded controlled environments, and thecorresponding system operating parameters (temperature, humidity and pressure differential).
7. Developing a detailed validation sampling plan satisfying all pertinent information requirements i.e., sample numbers and locations, time and date of samples, and the environment parameters (temperature, humidity and pressure differential).
8. Writing local Standard Operating Procedures for the routine operation, maintenance and monitoring of the controlled environments.
9. For new or upgraded controlled environments, a statement verifying that the controlled environments were constructed according to the approved blueprints and design specifications.

10. Developing the validation sampling plan and procedures
11. Collecting and assaying all validation samples as per requirements
12. Approving the results of the validation testing, including results of initial sample failures, retests and corresponding investigations.
13. Certifying the validation of the controlled environments.
14. Following the condition of new or upgraded controlled environments, submitting a set of as-built blueprints to EQA.
15. Notifying EQA of local regulatory requirements regarding validation.
16. Notifying EQA in writing of future design modifications, replacement of system components or changes in operating conditions, since these may require further validation testing.

C. Central Engineering, if involved in the construction of new or upgraded controlled environments, will be responsible for :

1. Notifying EQA in writing during the design phase of new or upgraded controlled environments
2. For new or upgraded controlled environments, submitting to EQA for approval draft blueprints and design specifications.
3. For new or upgraded controlled environments, submitting to EQA a final set of EQA approved blueprints and design specifications.
4. A statement verifying that the controlled environments were constructed according to the approved blueprints and design specifications.
5. Following the completion of new or upgraded controlled environments, submitting to EQA a final set of as-built blueprints.

Physical Criteria

1. Existing systems must meet the minimum design criteria for controlled environments in order to be considered for validation.
2. All newly constructed and installed controlled environments must meet the criteria listed in the Standards for Sterile Manufacturing and Sterility Testing. Any upgrades to existing systems must incorporate these standards.

Testing Criteria

Class 100 - sterile

Refers to the air environment of a designated area which is required to maintain a total particulate concentration of not greater than 25 particles/cu.ft (p/ft^3) in a size range of 0.5F and larger and a viable air concentration no greater than 1 Colony Forming Unit per cu. m (CFU/m^3) of air sampled during validation testing. Examples of a Class 100 environment are a laminar flow hood and a sterile filling line.

Class 10,000 - clean

Refers to the air environment of a designated area which is required to maintain a total particulate concentration of not greater than 2,500 particles/cu.ft (p/ft^3) in a size range of 0.5F and larger and a viable air concentration no greater than 2 Colony Forming Units per cu. m (CFU/m^3) of air sampled during validation testing. Examples of a Class 10,000 environment are an aseptic batching area, filling room or sterility testing room.

Class 100,000 - ancillary

Refers to the air environment of a designated area which is required to maintain a total particulate concentration of not greater than 25,000 particles/cu.ft (p/ft^3) in a size range of 0.5F and larger and a viable air concentration no greater than 5 Colony Forming Units per cu. m (CFU/m^3) of air sampled during validation testing. Examples of a Class 100,000 environment are a gowning area and airlock.

Validation Sampling Plan

Classification of Area	Size of Area (m^2)[1]	Number of Samples/location Work level		Air supply	
		P	**V**	**P**	**V**
Class 100	< 1	1	1	1	1
(Sterile)	1 to 3	3	3	2	2
Plus one additional sample at each location for every multiple of $3m^2$, or fraction thereof in excess of $3m^2$					
Class 10,000	< 10	1	1	1	1
(Clean)	10 to 20	2	2	1	1
	20 to 50	3	3	2	2
Plus one additional sample at each location for every multiple of $50m^2$, or fraction thereof in excess of $50m^2$					
Class 100,000	< 10	1	1	1	1
(Ancillary)	10 to 30	2	2	1	1
	30 to 80	3	3	2	2

Key to Superscript

1 m^2 for Class 100 refers to the total area of HEPA/ULPA filter face in the laminar flow module; for Class 10,000 and Class 100,000 it refers to the total area of the room.

Sampling conditions

1. The area to be validated must be sanitised with an appropriate disinfecting agent and the air system in continuous operation for a minimum of 24 hours prior to any sampling. Once the validation testing has begun, the system must operate for 24 hours per day, 7 days per week.
2. All sampling within the area to be validated will be performed under normal operational set up (such as the filling line and filling equipment), but in the absence of production activity. The only personnel present in the test area should be the validation samplers.
3. The area being validated must be operating under the same environmental conditions of temperature, humidity and pressure differentials as specified for normal operational activity. These parameters must be recorded during the period of validation testing.
4. DOP testing must have been performed and documented within the past twelve months.

Sampling criteria

1. Air viable samples will be collected using a New Brunswick Scientific Slit-to-Agar biological air sampler, or approved equivalent. Use TSA (tripticase soy agar or soybean-casein digest agar) media plates prepared in-house or commercially prepared.
2. All air viable and total particulate work level samples will be taken into the direction of the air supply at work activity level (the level of the bottle opening on the filling line, and at approximately 75-100 cm above the floor within a room).
3. All air viable and total particulate air supply samples will be taken into the direction of the air supply within 30 cm of the filter face, ceiling register or supply duct. Accessory sampling probes attached to the inlet of the sampling unit may be used for this purpose.
4. An air viable sample taken at either the air supply or the work level will consist of 2 cu m of air with the results expressed as the average number of Colony Forming Units per cu m (CFU/m^3) of air sampled.
5. A total particulate sample taken at either the air supply or work level will

consist of 10 cu ft of air and the results expressed as the average number of particles per cu ft (p/ft^3) of air sampled

Approval limits

Classification of Area	Average[1] Total Particulates P/ft^3	Air viable CFU/m^3
Class 100 (Sterile)	25	1
Class 10,000 (Clean)	2,500	2
Class 100,000 (Ancillary)	25,000	5

Key to superscript

1 Total average for all samples taken at either the air supply or work level.

7 Human Interface in Controlled Environments

A cleanroom is a special environment constructed at great cost, operated and maintained at great expense, with the sole purpose of insuring consistency in product quality and value and minimising product contamination or failure. The best design, layout and materials are worthless if the people working in the cleanroom do not fully understand its significance or the *whats* and *whys* of its operations.

Even in the best designed clean rooms microcontamination continues to occur, and research studies on causes of such occurrences reveal that in 8 out of 10 cases failure can be traced to the humans in the environment. It is

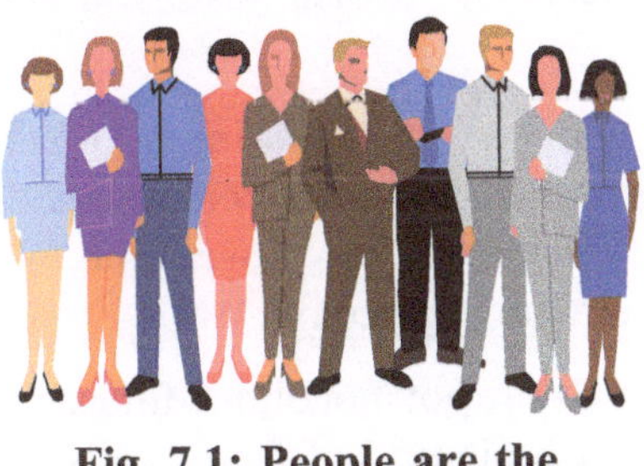

Fig. 7.1: People are the largest single source of contaminants in cleanrooms

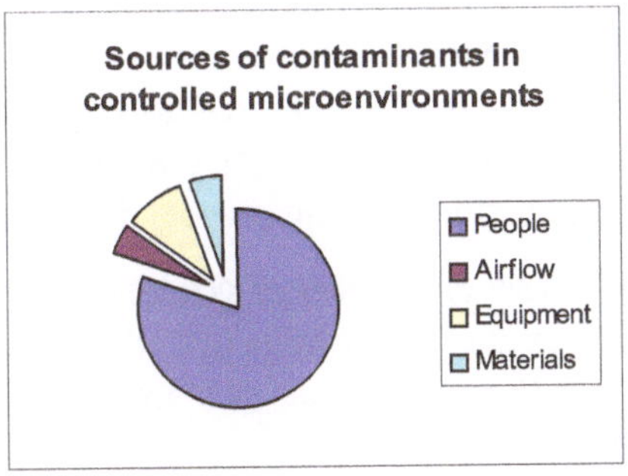

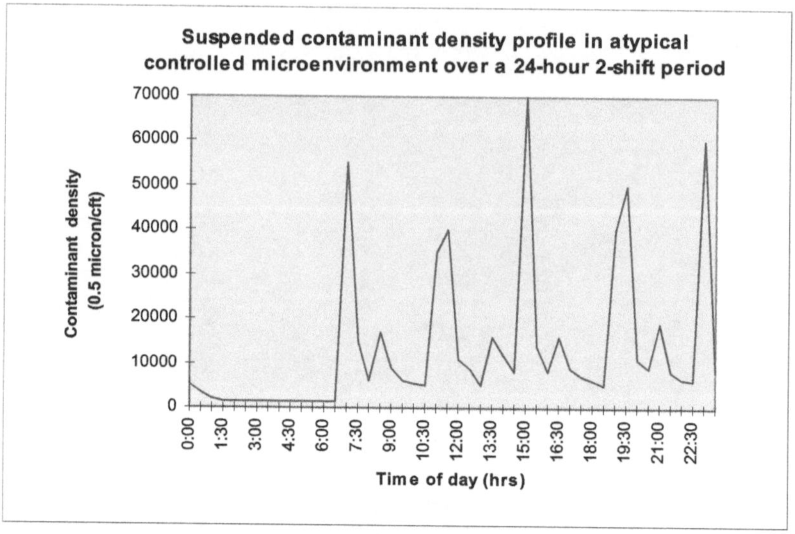

Fig. 7.2

common knowledge that contaminant level shoots up at commencement of shift, and is directly proportional to the number of people in the room. It drops only when activity ceases, and people exit.

With the employee brought into such sharp focus in the microcontamination control process, training in good manufacturing practices becomes one of the more important factors that influence the quality and consistency of the finished product. GMP is a responsibility that spans the organisation, and the people are its prime movers. The Orange Guide, WHO Guidelines and USFDA devote several paras to training and comportment, excerpts of which are reproduced here for ready reference.

Humans may be viewed as biologic factories. They take in food, water and air; generate energy; manufacture cells and other body parts for growth, repair or replacement; and produce by-products and wastes, just as in any common continuous processing plant.

Thus having a human in a cleanroom is in reality permitting a hi-tech functioning mobile bioprocessing plant into your environment, complete with its effluents. As part of our microcontamination control programme, we begin by studying this *factory* from the cleanroom perspective.

The several layers of skin that cover the body are not monolithic films, but an aggregate of millions of cells, each a microscopic fig leaf. These cells die as a matter of course, and are constantly replenished. This includes scalp flakes, or dandruff.

Orange Guide 2002: Annexure 1

Para 14: *All personnel (including those concerned with cleaning and maintenance) exployed in such areas should receive regular training in disciplines relevant to the correct manufacture of sterile products. The training should include reference to hygiene and to the basic elements of microbiology. When outside staff who have not received such training (eg. building or maintenance contractors) need to be brought in, particular care should be taken over their instruction and supervision.*

Para 15: Staff who have been engaged in the processing of animal tissue materials or of cultures of microorganisms other than used in the current manufacturing process should not enter sterile product areas unless rigorous and clearly defined entry procedures have been followed.

Para 16: High standards of personal hygiene and cleanliness are essential. Personnel involved in the manufacture of sterile preparations should be instructed to report any condition which may cause the shedding of abnormal numbers or types of contaminants; periodic health checks for such for such conditions are desirable. Actions to be taken about personnel who could be introducing undue microbiological hazard should be decided by a designated competent person.

Annexure 18, Para 3.12: Training should be regularly conducted by qualified individualsand should cover, at a minimum, the particular operations that the employee performs and GMP as it relates to the employee's functions. Records of training should be maintained. Training should be periodically assessed.

WHO 2002: Main Principles: Para 10.4: All personnel should be aware of the principles of GMP that affect them and receive initial and continuing training...

Para 10.11: The manufacturer should provide training in accordance with a written programme for all the personnel whose duties take them into production areas or into control laboratories (including the technical, maintenance and cleaning personnel), and for other personnel whose activities could affect the quality of the product.

Para 10.12: Besides basic training on the theory and practice of GMP, newly recruited personnelshould receive training appropriate to the duties assigned to them. Continuing training should also be given, and its practical effectiveness should also be assessed. Training programmes should be available, approved by the head of either production or quality control, as appropriate. Training records should be kept.

Section 211.25, Personnel Qualifications requires that "each person engaged in manufacture, processing, packing or holding of a drug product shall have education, training and experience, or any combination thereof, to enable that person to perform the assigned functions ...Each person responsible for supervising the manufacture, processing, packing, or holding of a drug product shall have the education, training, and experience, or any combination thereof, to perform assigned functions in such a manner as to provide assurance that the drug product has the safety, identity, strength, quality, and purity that it purports or is represented to possess."

Section 211.25 also requires that continuing training in CGMP "shall be conducted by qualified individuals on a continuing basis and with sufficient frequency to assure that employees remain familiar with CGMP requirements applicable to them." The training "shall be in the particular operations that the employee performs and in current good manufacturing practice (including the current good manufacturing practice regulations in this chapter and written procedures required by these regulations), as they relate to the employee's functions."

Draft USFDA Guidelines for Sterile Drug Products Produced by Aseptic Processing:

Appropriate training should be conducted before an individual is permitted to enter the aseptic processing area and perform operations. For example, such training should include aseptic technique, clean room behavior, microbiology, hygiene, gowning, and patient safety hazard posed by a non-sterile drug product, and the specific written procedures covering aseptic processing area operations. After initial training, personnel should be updated regularly by an ongoing training program.

Personnel can have substantial impact on the quality of the environment in which the sterile product is processed. A vigilant and responsive personnel monitoring program should be established. Monitoring should be accomplished by obtaining surface samples of each aseptic processing operator's gloves on an at least a daily basis, or in association with each batch. This sampling should be accompanied by an appropriate sampling frequency for other strategically selected locations of the gown. The quality control unit should establish a more comprehensive monitoring program for operators involved in operations which are especially labor intensive, i.e. those requiring repeated or complex aseptic manipulations.

Asepsis is fundamental to an aseptic processing operation. An ongoing goal for manufacturing personnel in the aseptic processing room is to maintain contamination-free gloves throughout operations.

When operators exceed established levels or show an adverse trend, an investigation should be conducted promptly. Follow-up actions may include increased sampling, increased observation, retraining, gowning requalification, and in certain instances, reassignment of the individual to operations outside of the aseptic processing area.

These dead cells are continually discarded. Unlike trees, which shed leaves only in one season, our skin cells are shed every minute of every living day and night. These cells are approximately 30μ in length, 5μ in width and less than 0.5μ in thickness. The rate at which skin cells are shed is influenced by the condition of the skin, its oil content, the climate and the nature of activity. After shave lotions dissolve skin oils and accelerate sloughing and flaking. Similarly, alcohols, while popular as disinfectants, unless used with emollients like glycerol, tend to dissolve the skin oils and aggravate shedding. Austin and others have carried out extensive studies on this phenomenon and their results are summarised here.

The different organisms present on the skin may be classified as *transient* organisms (microorganisms which are deposited on and contaminate the skin but do not multiply there), *temporary residents* (viable contaminants that multiply on the skin and persist for short periods) and *resident* organisms (microorganisms which colonise the deeper crevices of the skin and hair follicles - 20% of skin bacteria are situated deep within the skin, covered and protected by lipids and superficial cornified epithelium, and are most inaccessible). The numbers and types of bacteria on the skin differ considerably according to the body site where they are found, or the sampling technique that may be employed. In addition, individual variation in numbers is vast. This variation can depend upon skin pH, fatty acids, age, condition, and the temperature and humidity of the skin and environment. Some people may spread bacteria more easily than others. Although the number of bacteria on the skin of the hand is comparatively low, there is still a wide variation from person to person. It is known that some individuals have consistently high bacterial counts on their finger tips, while others have very low counts regardless of the method of hand washing or disinfectant employed. Swabs are increasingly being taken from parts of the body other than the conventional glove/finger prints. One organisation takes swab samples from soles of operators' feet, abdomen, forearm and forehead.

While it is generally agreed that the removal or killing of the transient and temporarily resident flora is sufficient to prevent their transfer to the product, any removal of resident flora is deemed a valuable additional safeguard.

The body has glands all over, each producing its own substance. Oils, sweat, saline, saliva, and wax are some of the substances so produced that have the potential to contaminate the environment. We are familiar with the oil stains that accompany our finger prints; each time we blink we splash saline; when we open our mouths we spray droplets of saliva; the sweat we generate passes through our clothes to a greater or lesser extent, depending on the permeability of the fabric, by capillary action; on evaporation of sweat the residual salts remain deposited on our skin cells. Chlorides of sodium and potassium are routinely found on analysing the contaminants in clean rooms.

Hair becomes statically charged on combing, and attracts dust. Oiled hair retains the dust better than dry hair. Dry hair is brittle and breaks easily. Hair also produces a protein called keratanin, which is released into the environment.

Studies indicate that a man on an average breathes 16,000 quartz of air per day, which converts to approximately 20 kg/day! And this aerosol is exhaled from a distance as close as 20 to 40 cms from the sensitive work piece. Inhalation disturbs the air pattern around the work area; exhalation carries a mixture of gases, vapour, liquid droplets, mucous and, of course,

Table 7.1: Austin's Index of contaminants shed by personnel

Activity	Particles ≥ 0.3μ emitted per minute	Viable contaminants generated per minute
Standing or sitting without movement	100,000	750
Light head, hand & forearm movement	500,000	1,000
Moderate body and arm movement	1,000,000	1,500
Changing positions - sitting to standing	2,500,000	2,500
Slow walking	5,000,000	4,000
Moderate walking	7,500,000	8,000
Fast walking	10,000,000	15,000
Climbing stairs	10,000,000	15,000
Calisthenics	≥ 15,000,000	30,000
Coughing	≥ 15,000,000	≥ 30,000
Sneezing (excluding large droplets)	≥ 30,000,000	≥ 50,000

microorganisms. In particular, the exhaled air is rich with dust and other allergens that the lung is anxious to be rid of, and such contaminants are often thrown out with unusual force. Extreme examples are coughs and sneezes.

Smokers breathe out more contaminants than nonsmokers, even several hours after they have last smoked. Drinking water after smoking helps slightly reduce the number exhaled.

Cuts, abrasions, wounds, rashes, allergies and boils; and topical medicaments, dressings and plasters further aggravate the problem. Other

Table 7.2: Human Bioprofile

Site	Aerobic flora		Anaerobic flora	
	Males	Females	Males	Females
Forehead	2075	1225	8000	13500
Sternum	2125	165	50000	3500
Subclavicular area	350	130	18500	2275
Centre back	450	155	67500	7500
Shoulder	128	48	1025	1075
Deltoid area	118	65	57	127
Forearm	250	35	9	13
Palm	98	155	33	85
Lower axilla	500	92	14	12
Lumbar area	300	33	178	142
Periumblical area	850	175	55	80
Thigh upper front	325	140	9	35
Thigh lower front	350	67	14	16
Thigh back	325	82	4	5
Shin	190	77	7	8
Calf	173	20	2	5
Dorsum of foot	80	122	3	10
Sole	22750	675	10	4

conditions requiring care and vigil are discharges from eyes, ears, and nose; coughs, colds and sneezes; and, of course, menstrual periods.

Body temperature is maintained at 37 ^{0}C; but the skin temperature varies from head to toe as can be demonstrated by thermographic techniques. The average of these values is usually around 33 ^{0}C. Since the cleanroom is designed to operate within the range 22 - 24 ^{0}C, the body surface is at an average of about 10 ^{0}C above its surroundings. This thermal gradient triggers convective currents rising from floor level to above the head. These currents disturb the airflow pattern in the room.

These are some of the *intrinsic* contaminants ushered in with every human being who enters the cleanroom. Once we understand the body and its danger zones, it is easier to devise ways and means to contain the damage they can cause.

Not only do people produce contaminants, but they also serve as unwitting carriers of contaminants that are *extrinsic* to them. Starting from the water they wash with; the soaps they use; the towels and napkins; the undergarments and street clothes; the cosmetics and makeup; jewellery and personal

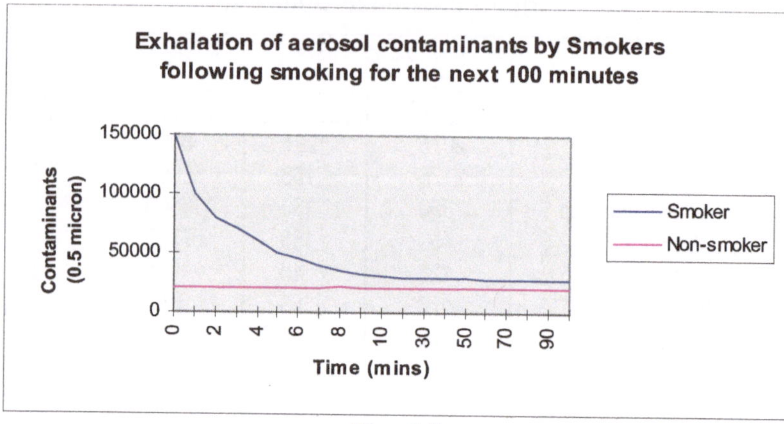

Fig. 7.3

effects -all these make their contributions to the contaminant load carried by the individual. Analysis of the contaminants found in clean rooms show compounds of zinc and magnesium and talc, all originating from the talcum powders used by both men and women.

The dust and grit on the streets, the grime and soot in the air; the jostling in crowds while they commute to work covers them all over with potential contaminants. And since people are mobile, they carry these contaminants with them wherever they go, leaving a trail along their path and place in jeopardy whatever they handle or touch. Movement also causes disturbance in the airflow field, and depending on how they move, they cause turbulence and eddies in their wake of varying severity. The greater the number of people in a room, the higher the contaminant level, and greater the risk of product contamination.

Now that we know about the human microenvironment, and how humans can be vectors of contaminants, we can devise ways and means to control, if not altogether stop contamination from occurring.

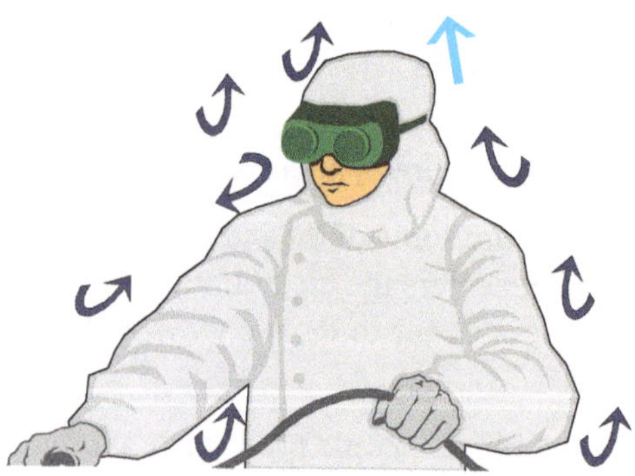

Fig. 7.4: Convection currents around the human body

Good Gowning Practice

Garments should be worn correctly to serve the intended purpose. The gowning procedure described here is intended to serve as a guide; you should draw up your own gowning sequence by modifying this procedure wherever necessary.

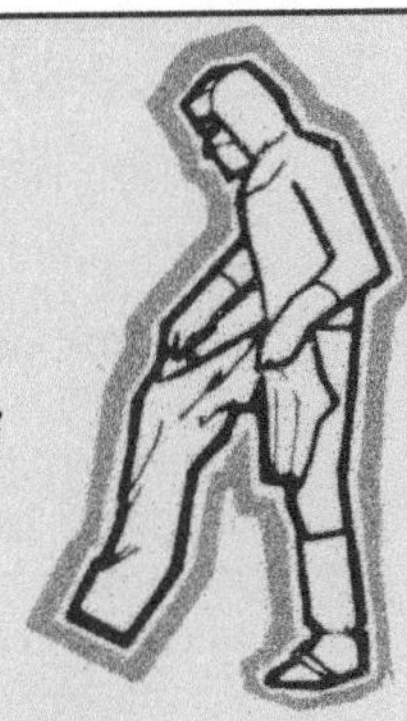

- Remove street footwear. Change into cleanroom footwear.
- Remove all street garments not necessary for warmth or modesty
- Remove and safely store watches, rings, cigarettes, lighters, jewellery, purse and other personal effects.
- Scrub down. Remove cosmetics, if any applied. Use appropriate cleanroom grade detergent compatible with the disinfectants used to remove physical contaminants.
- Washing of hands and forearms deserves special care. The under surfaces of finger nails should be thoroughly cleaned with a soft nylon brush, or when necessary, with a scraper.
- Wear gowning cap. This is optional at this point in the gowning sequence. The purpose is to conceal the hair at an early stage, and keep it covered thereafter.
- Enter change room. Installation of a good quality "tacky" mat at entrance is recommended. If you are not sure of the quality, you are better off without it. Even with a good tacky mat, research has established that you need to walk a distance of 20 steps before you have left behind 95% of your footborne debris. Having a "Welcome" size tacky mat may not be as useful as imagined.
- Wear gowning gloves. This is also optional at this stage. The objective is to avoid contact with washed bare hands. Select gloves of proper style and size.

- Carefully put on the first glove, touching the outside of the glove as little as possible. Then put on the second glove, taking care not to touch anything other than cleanroom apparel.
- Obtain cleanroom apparel and accessories appropriate for your task and prepare for donning.
- The first item to be worn is the legwear. Inspect the item for damages and stains and once satisfied sit on the "barrier" stool, if available, or on a chair or bench, and put on the first boot, taking care to ensure that it does not touch the floor. Then swing the *clean* foot over to the cleanroom side of the stool or bench.Put on the second boot and swing over fully to the cleanroom side and stand up.
- Next put on your head cover, if necessary over the cap already on. Adjust to cover hair fully. Take care not to touch anything other than the items of garments.
- Put on face mask, where applicable.
- Now prepare the coverall for wearing it. Inspect for tears and soil, keeping it off the floor. Step into legs and then pull on the upper half. Tuck the skirt of the hood inside the collar of the coverall or coat. Close all fasteners at neck and wrists. Tuck legs of garment into boots and refasten legwear till it is snug and comfortable.
- Discard gowning gloves, if worn. Disinfect hands as per procedure prescribed by your SOP. Put on working gloves using the same technique and care described earlier for donning gloves. Tuck cuffs of garment into gloves.
- Check that all leg, and arm openings are completely sealed with gloves and boots.
- Do not adjust garment after donning working gloves. As a matter of fact your gloved hand should now touch only your work related objects and nothing else.
- Proceed through air shower and across another tacky mat to enter the cleanroom.

The first regulation begins with ascertaining the bare minimum number of people the cleanroom requires and setting the limit on the head count in the room on this basis and declaring the area out of bounds for others. In addition to restricting the entry into the cleanroom, there should be further restrictions for accessing critical environments within the cleanroom itself.

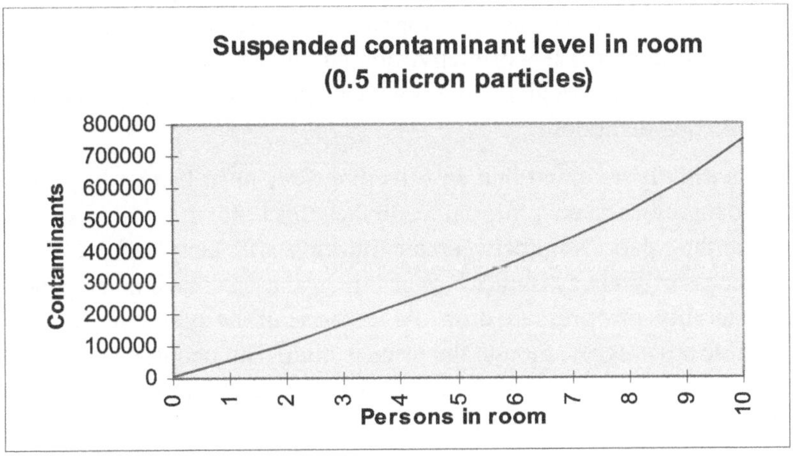

Fig. 7.5

Decontamination procedures prior to entry should be clearly enunciated and strictly enforced. Gowning procedures should be drawn up to suit the requirements of the environment cleanliness aspired. Once finalised, these procedures must be rigidly adhered to.

Since behaviour is so important, industrial engineering techniques of time and motion study should be applied while drawing up the overall personnel flow chart, with emphasis on reducing personnel movements and body actions to minimal levels for optimal performance. The operating procedures so arrived at should form the base for rigorous training in operation skills imparted to employees.

Selection of Contamination Control Clothing : Anyone in the cleanroom business who wants an argument need only mention the term *garment.* To many it is much like religion - they already know what they believe, and no mere *fact* can ever change their minds. We are assuming that there are at least some people who may be interested in looking at the evidence and want to take a fresh look at the parameters of concern. We cannot decide for you; but we can cover the aspects to consider when a decision must be made.

The objective function of contamination control clothing is to serve as a barrier between the human microenvironment and the cleanroom, keeping particulates, skin flakes and the like from the operator from escaping into the cleanroom environment. In effect the garment is a filter. This garment/filter system must allow air and moisture to flow through and carry off heat and moisture generated by the wearer. Ideally a rubber bag or plastic suiting would be an excellent system for stopping the contaminants, but would be a poor garment in any real-world environment, and the final choice is often a trade off between the ideal and the practical, since the wearer's comfort is an important consideration.

It is normally assumed that an effective filter must have a high pressure drop, and therefore be uncomfortable. In fact, this is not the case. Experiments show that the relationship between air filtration efficiency and pressure drop is not necessarily always linear. What we want is a reasonably good filter with a tolerably low pressure drop. At least one of the synthetics, DACRON, offers these advantages, though the price is high. But economising on gowns can prove costly beyond estimation: and compromising on clothing quality can place your product and reputation at high risk.

All the Guidelines for Good Manufacturing Practice speak with one voice on the importance of good gowning practice.

The first consideration, therefore, is the choice of the fabric itself. The important characteristics to look for are that it should not lint; it should at least not generate static charges; should be fire-retardant if not flameproof; and should be treated for water repellency and inhibition of microbial growth. Conductive fabrics are fully effective only when connected through conductive wrist straps and controlled resistance to ground. Otherwise, they are only sub-optimally effective. Such fabrics are recommended mainly where ESD or static induced fire and/or explosions are concerns.

Some applications are more sensitive to static charge dissipation than others, determined by the susceptibility of the product (microelectronic) or the environment (vulnerable to explosions). These applications demand conductive fabrics where electrically conductive fibres (carbon filament or carbon treated polyamide filament) is woven together with DACRON filaments resulting in strict electrostatic and particulate protection without any external or chemical treatments. (The best chemically treated fibres lose their conductive properties progressively with each successive wash). Such fabrics effectively prevent electrostatic surges by means of constant, rapid and controlled dissipation of charges (positive or negative) through low level ionisation or corona discharge to the atmosphere. A fabric is deemed to be antistatic if its surface resistivity

Table 7.3: Recommended selection and usage of garments

Class	M / E	#M2.5 / #10	M3.5 / 100	M4.5 / 1,000	M5.5 / 10,000	M6.5 / 100,000
Items		Coverall Hood Mask Boots Gloves	Coverall Hood Boots Gloves	Coverall or Coat Hood Overshoes Gloves	Lab coat Cap Overshoes	Lab coat Cap Overshoes
Change		Per entry	Daily	Daily	3/week	2/week

Table 7.4: Cleanroom fabric characteristics

Parameter	Conductive*	Non-static
Composition	99% DACRON+ 1% CARBON texsq continuous mono filament polymer yarn Taffetta style weave	100% DACRON 150d or 50% DACRON 85d 50% NOMEX 40TL texsq polymeric blend in Taffeta or Herring bone style weave
Lint character	non-linting	non-linting
Weight	125 gms/sq m	68 - 90 gm/sq m
Weave	30 x 30/sq cm	30 x 25/sq cm
Break strength	25 Kg/25 mm width	25 Kg/25 mm width
Elongation	80% of rupture	80% of rupture
Resistivity	10^6 - 10^{10}ohms/sq cm	13 x 10^{14} ohms/sq cm
Voltage decay	1/10 sec 90% 1 sec 100%	1/2 sec 72% 40 sec 90%
Static character	conductive	non-static
Chemical	Resists acid	Resists acid/alkali
Permeability	0.00022 - 0.001 mps 100 cum/hr/sq m @ 25 mm wc	0.005 - 0.035 mps 100 cum/hr/sq m @ 25 mm wc
Efficiency	89% down to 0.5 μ 100% down to 5.0 μ	82% down to 0.5 μ 100% down to 5.0 μ
Durability	200 cycles	200 cycles
Taber abrasion (% fibre loss)	0.3% (unlaundered)	0.6% (unlaundered)

* *Fully effective only when connected through conductive wrist straps and controlled resistance to ground. Otherwise, only sub-optimally effective. Recommended mainly where ESD or static induced fire or explosion are concerns*

is 10^{11} ohms per square centimetre or lower; conductive fabrics have resistivities in the range 10^6 to 10^9. Uniformly distributed and controlled electrostatic discharge ensures cleaner fabric surface, improves personal comfort and offers greater protection to the product, environment and the operator.

After you have selected the fabric, you decide on the patterns that best suit your needs, and award the conversion contract to an agency that is familiar with the special care required for tailoring contamination control clothing. Cut edges should be heat-sealed; stitching should be double-seamed; tailoring should ensure that no raw edges are exposed and that there are no collection points where dirt and lint can be deposited and accumulated. As a general rule, pockets and belts must be avoided.

Errors in gowning are common, and often negate the very purpose of wearing contamination control apparel. Exposing or improperly covering hair, face, moustaches and beards, wrists, street clothing, ankles and street shoes should be scrupulously avoided. Even after gowning, some contaminants do escape into the environment, but the numbers are greatly reduced.

To derive the maximum protection offered by contamination control clothing, special care is needed in the manner, as well as the environment in which it is washed, dried, pressed and packed. It is unfortunately common to find cleanroom clothing sent out for laundering. It is paradoxical: so much care is taken in selection and procurement of these clothes; but little thought is spared to reflect on what is needed for cleaning them after every use. The local laundry was not designed to handle such garments, and the environment there is bound to be anything but dust-free.

Orange Guide 2002 Annexure 1 Para 21 addresses this concern, and strongly advocates the setting up of a dedicated in-house laundering facility.

The complete procedure described here is for your guidance. Setting up an in-house laundry, close to the main cleanroom, offers advantages you cannot ignore. The cleanroom laundry air cleanliness level could be one class lower than that being maintained in the processing area and the regulations enforced there should apply to the laundry too.

After entry decontamination and gowning, we have one more device at our disposal to minimise the probability of contamination: generate as little as possible within the cleanroom. This demands *good conduct and strict discipline.*

Again, all the Guidelines urge training in proper comportment and conduct within sterile preparation areas. For example, the Draft USFDA Guideline devotes a whole section on personnel, and has this to say:

Fig. 7.6: Washing soiled contamination control apparel

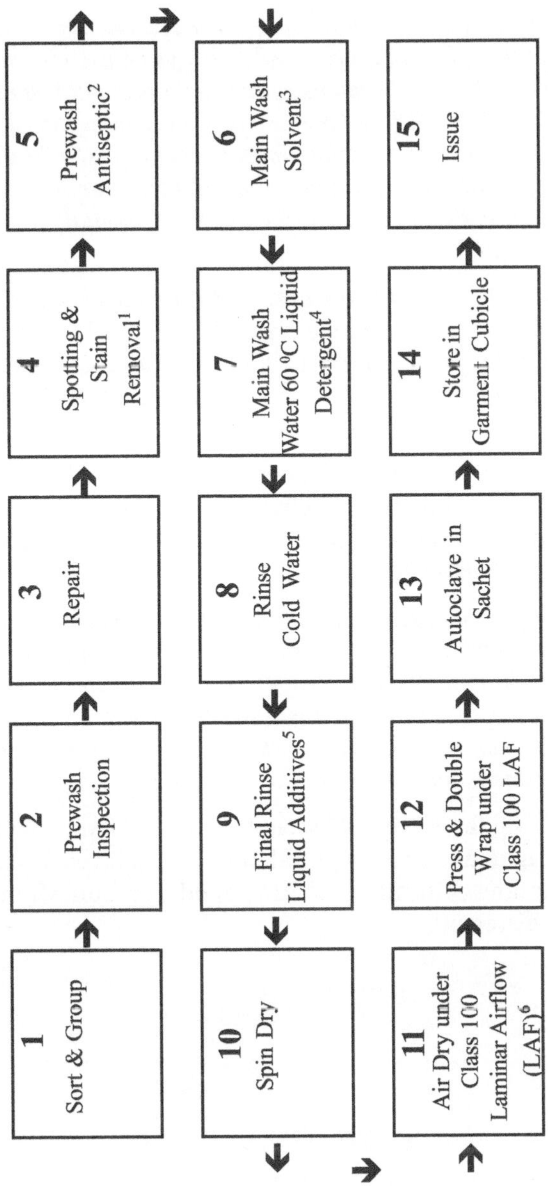

1. Hyglo, Teepol, Clinitol, or CCl_4
2. Savlon, Dettol/Iteol, Hydrogen peroxide or Peracetic acid
3. Perchloroethylene, Trichloroethylene or Mineral turpentine
4. Ezee, or Genteel
5. Antistatic agent, Optical whitener, Fabric softener (Carboxymethyl cellulose 5% v/v)
6. Class M6.5 (100,000) or better

Adherence to basic aseptic technique is a continuous requirement for operators in an aseptic processing operation. Some of these techniques aimed at maintaining sterility of sterile items and surfaces include :

1. *Contacting sterile materials only with sterile instruments. Sterile instruments (e.g., forceps) are should always be used in the handling of sterilized materials. Between uses, instruments should be placed only in sterilized containers. These instruments should be replaced as necessary throughout the operation. After initial gowning, sterile gloves should be regularly sanitized to minimize the risk of contamination. Personnel should not directly contact sterile products, containers, closures, or critical surfaces.*

2. *Moving slowly and deliberately. Rapid movements can create unacceptable turbulence in the critical zone. Such movements disrupt the sterile field, presenting a challenge beyond intended cleanroom design and control parameters. The principle of slow, careful movement should be followed throughout the cleanroom.*

3. *Keeping the entire body out of the path of laminar air. Laminar airflow design is used to protect sterile equipment surfaces, container-closures, and product. Personnel should not disrupt the path of laminar flow air in the aseptic processing zone.*

4. *Approaching a necessary manipulation in a manner that does not compromise sterility of the product. In order to maintain sterility of nearby sterile materials, a proper aseptic manipulation should be approached from the side and not above the product (in vertical laminar flow operations). Also, speaking when in direct proximity to an aseptic processing line is not an acceptable practice.*

Posters explaining the *Whats, Whys* and *Hows* of Good Aseptic Practices drawn up with imagination and wit and should be displayed at vantage points to serve as constant reminders of the need for compliance and the consequences of disregard.

8 Cleaning Cleanrooms

The purpose of cleaning is to remove soil, any substance that is not an integral part of a structure, or designed to assist in function. This objective may be modified by practicality and cost, and should be achieved without shortening the life of the item, interfering with its function, or increasing the risk of contamination. Any item after cleaning should have fewer rather than more contaminants on it. Contaminated water, soiled mops or wipes often increase the number of viable and nonviable contaminants on a surface. The source of soil may be particles deposited from the air or transferred by direct contact from hands, equipment or implements.

Soil removal is not merely to prevent it from contaminating a product, though it is certainly the single most important objective in the context of aseptic zones. Soil can obliterate identification marks, warnings or instructions on equipment; corrode, abrade or react chemically with a surface; block channels, interfere with valves, or the flow of liquids, gases or electric current; encourage insects, pests or growth of microorganisms; form an insulating shield that obstructs penetration of heat or chemicals, specially during sterilisation or disinfection; and can generally reduce the confidence in the facility's ability to deliver quality products.

Aseptic Zone Cleaning

Aseptic zone cleaning is a specialised task, which requires trained staff that will keep to detailed schedules, and often requires equipment, methods and materials not used in other situations. Why? Because soil in aseptic zones can potentiate product contamination. To add to our difficulties, the bulk of the contaminants encountered in aseptic zones are invisible. How do you clean what you cannot see?

If we have gravel or river sand soiling our clothes, we merely shake it off, or brush it off. But if red mud or talcum powder gets on our clothes, we find it more difficult to dislodge it. Washing with water usually solves the problem. If some paint or blood stain soils our clothes it takes more than soap and water to remove the stains.

This is because particles, like gravel, in the size range above 20μ do not bond strongly with the surface they are in contact, and can be removed by conventional methods employing simple brushing or detergents and water. This is primary or gross cleaning.

Particles, like fine mud or talc, in the size range of 0.1μ to 20μ are influenced by considerations like polarity and surface tension, and require coaxing with surfactants (surface acting agents) for removal. This constitutes secondary or precision cleaning.

Particles, like stains, in the size range below 0.1μ bond aggressively through forces of intermolecular attraction, and can be persuaded only by strong solvents. This is tertiary cleaning or cleansing.

Analogies from our day-to-day cleaning experiences: gross cleaning while dusting, sweeping and wiping; moderate precision cleaning while bathing, washing clothes and polishing articles; and tertiary cleaning while removing stains.

Whether it is an aseptic zone floor or ceiling, work surface or component, equipment or tool, it is necessary that we identify the nature of the contaminant and choose a cleaning technique appropriate for that task.

Methods of Cleaning

Two basic methods of cleaning are used: dry and wet. Dry methods rely on mechanical action to loosen and remove larger objects and particulate soil, but do not remove stains and are unsuitable for wet, oily or greasy surfaces. Wet cleaning employs detergent solutions, surfactants and solvents to loosen and resuspend or dissolve adherent soil.

Table 8.1: Cleanroom soil characteristics

	Diameter of particles (microns)	Velocity of Settling: *Feet per minute*	*Inches per hour*	*Centimeters per Second*		
Tertiary cleaning	< 0.02	?	?	?	Brownian-Van der Waal Regime	Diffusion
Secondary cleaning	0.05	0.00003	0.022	0.000015	Uncertainty Regime	Drag
	0.1	0.00016	0.115	0.000081		
	0.2	0.00036	0.259	0.00018		
	0.4	0.0013	0.936	0.00066		
	0.8	0.005	3.6	0.0025		
	1	0.007	5.04	0.0036		
	2	0.024	17.4	0.012		
	5	0.2	144	0.102		
	10	0.59	425	0.3		
Primary cleaning	20	2.4	1,728	1.2	Newtonian Regime	Gravity
	40	9.5	6,840	4.8		
	60	21.3	15,320	10.8		
	80	37.9	27,250	19.2		
	100	352	253,500	179		
	400	498	360,000	253		

Clean is a relative concept; and attempting to clean soil too small to be seen adds to the challenge of good cleanroom housekeeping.

Particles in the gravitational regime (20µ and larger) do not bond strongly with the surface they are in contact, and can be removed by conventional methods employing detergents and water. This is primary or gross cleaning.

Particles in the drag regime are influenced by considerations like polarity and surface tension, and require coaxing with surfactants (surface acting agents) for removal. This constitutes secondary or precision cleaning. Particles in the diffusion regime bond aggressively through forces of intermolecular attraction, and can be persuaded only by strong solvents. This is tertiary cleaning or cleansing.

Cleaning Cleanrooms

- ***Two basic methods of cleaning are used: dry and wet. Dry methods rely on mechanical action to loosen and remove larger objects and particulate soil, but do not remove stains and are unsuitable for wet, oily or greasy surfaces. Wet cleaning employs detergent solutions, surfactants and solvents to loosen and resuspend or dissolve adherent soil.***

- ***Cleaning should not be an exercise in redistribution of soil or cause increase of suspendedcontaminants***

Sweeping	*700%*	*increase*
Dust attracting mop	*30%*	*increase*
Wet scrubbing machines	*3%*	*increase*
Vacuum without filter	*25%*	*increase*
Vacuum with HEPA	*20%*	*decrease*

- ***All locations in a cleanroom do not generate the same volume of soil***

- ***Staging area for pre-entry decontamination protocols help reduce the burden within.***

- ***Cleanroom practices adopted during installation. (Cleanroom Construction Protocol) keeps background count low at start up***

Cleaning should not end up as an exercise in redistribution of settled contaminants. For example, sweeping with brooms increases suspended contaminant density by 700%! Dust attracting mops cause an increase of 30%; wet scrubbing machines by 3%. Vacuum cleaning without filtered exhaust increases the count by 25%; if fitted with a HEPA exhaust, it causes a decrease in the count by 20%. The effect varies with the make of equipment and manner of use.

Hazards while Cleaning

Cleaning should not be undertaken while the aseptic zone is in operation; if unavoidable, first cover all susceptible sites and open vessels and allow at least 15 minutes for dispersed contaminants to settle out of harm's way before re-exposing them. Though dispersal of contaminants into the air is less likely with wet cleaning, the solutions become contaminated quickly; splashes are common, and aerosol droplets can travel far and wide to contaminate. Wet methods require proper drying out after the cleaning process; otherwise they bring in their own store of problems like accelerated microbial growth, corrosion and chemical attacks, and slippery floors. Besides, if a detergent or soap is used for cleaning, it is important to consider the difficulty that may arise with build up of residues, which must be deemed as yet another type of soil.

Detergents and their Residues

A common problem associated with detergents is its composition. Suppliers do not provide specific data on composition, which makes it difficult to evaluate residues. Unlike product residues, where tolerance levels for residual concentration are often laid down and accepted, there are no corresponding acceptance limits for detergent residues, since detergents are not part of the manufacturing process and are added only to facilitate the cleaning process. If the detergent is not easily removable, a different, more suitable detergent should be selected.

Detergents and their Residues

A common problem associated with detergents is its composition. Suppliers do not provide specific data on composition, which makes it difficult to evaluate residues. Unlike product residues, where tolerance levels for residual concentration are often laid down and accepted, there are no corresponding acceptance limits for detergent residues, since detergents are not part of the manufacturing process and are added only to facilitate the cleaning process. If the detergent is not easily removable, a different, more suitable detergent should be selected.

When in Doubt, Deem it Dirty

Some areas, by the nature of the function carried out there, may be heavily contaminated. While every effort is made to keep these areas as clean as possible, it is often more prudent to deem them as contaminated and take necessary precautions, rather than adopt expensive ineffective measures and then ignore the risk.

Setting up a Staging Area

There would be much less to clean down inside the aseptic zone if we were to make sure that all men and materials are sent in thoroughly cleaned. It is good practice to set up a staging area just outside the aseptic zone for carrying out final gross clean down prior to entry. If the equipment or component is manufactured under clean conditions; and if every item entering the aseptic zone is sent double-wrapped, so that the outer jacket serves as a dust cover and can be stripped in the staging area, the decontamination work load is reduced and the whole process becomes more effective.

In fact, aseptic zone practices are being increasingly adopted by cleanroom contractors while setting up an aseptic processing zone. Cleanroom Construction Protocol (discussed in Chapter 3) requires immediate pick up of spills; vacuuming while drilling; providing temporary curtains around site where

Cleaning Agents
Criteria for Selection

1. **Surface tension**
2. **Polarity**
3. **pH**
4. **Stability**
5. **Solubility**
6. **Reactivity**
7. **Efficiency as surfactant**
8. **Recommended use volume/unit surface area, dilution levels and temperature**
9. **Residue forming propensities**

dust generating operations are being carried out to avoid dispersal and spread of debris. Such techniques reduce the start up contaminant load, resulting in faster clean down on commissioning.

Cleaning Cleanrooms

- ***Cleaning should be introduced as a properly planned, coordinated and adequately researched programme***
- ***Choose a cleaning technique appropriate for the intended task***
- ***Microbial purity of water for cleaning should meet PHS standards, not more than 500 CFU/ml. Final rinse is recommended with pure water (WFI grade) containing not more than 100 CFU/ml at a temperature of 80 °C.***
- ***Because some equipment are very complex, chemical tests may be required to monitor residual detergents in the rinse water, and rinsing continued until the level falls below maximum acceptable limits. Where possible, drying should be under LAF cover.***
- ***The sanitation programme must take into account waste management***
  - ***What is to be collected***
  - ***What quantities are expected***
  - ***How must the waste be moved through and out of the area to prevent accumulation an d possible contamination***
  - ***How must the material be disposed off: municipal sewage, landfill or incineration***

Drawing up a Cleaning Programme

The first important step is to appoint a Contamination Control Team. Routine cleaning should be carried out as part of an agreed programme with detailed agreed schedules and procedures. Regimen drawn up for the facility should be given preference where it conflicts with the manufacturer's instructions, but it is always a good idea to read the instructions first and clarify discrepancies. Alternate methods or materials should not be used unless authorised. Cleaning products should not be mixed unless known to be compatible. Soaps and detergents may often reduce the effectiveness of disinfectants; some products may react dangerously. For example, soap neutralises quarternary ammonium compounds (like Savlon) and acid cleaners react on exposure to hypo chlorites (bleach) to release chlorine. Surface deterioration is often attributable to inappropriate cleaning. Not all commonly used cleaning techniques have been introduced as properly planned, coordinated and adequately researched programmes, and it is reasonable to check methods, which do not appear to be soundly based. It is part of the job of the contamination control team to liaise with other disciplines in evaluating the need for changes in existing procedures and programmes related to contamination risk.

Waste Management

The programme must provide for management of wastes. Waste includes spillage, defective packaging materials, containers and products. Estimates should be made of waste, both quantities and characteristics at various points in the manufacturing process and means of collection and disposal provided. The wastes must be effectively separated from the process stream to provide positive assurance that the product will not be contaminated. Disposal means, whether waste containers, dust collection equipment, vacuum collectors or even separate sewage system, should be clearly marked.

To illustrate the need to identify and separate waste streams, consider the liquid waste discharge from a pharmaceutical facility. The rest room, lavatory, and kitchen waste, known as domestic sanitary sewage, is one type; rinse water from process areas, tank drainage from compounding areas and laboratory wastes, known as industrial waste, is the other type. While the former may be directly discharged into a sanitary sewage system, the latter may require some pretreatment prior to discharge. To facilitate the streams, most production facilities have multiple sewage systems. This need to separate the two types of liquid waste streams is intended for the protection of the municipal sewage treatment system and facility.

Internally, the separation of process waste from domestic waste is necessary to help maintain the controlled conditions in the aseptic zone. If all liquid wastes were discharged via a single system, any blockage or overflow condition in that system could cause a overflow of one type of waste into the other, and domestic waste may find its way into the production area, introducing an unacceptable and indeterminate bacterial contamination. To preclude the possibility of this condition, pharmaceutical facilities have separate domestic and process waste systems, which do not connect with the plant, and are equipped to prevent backflow of waste into the facility.

Control of the waste disposal problem then involves a three-element system: solid waste disposal; liquid waste disposal; and airborne waste (dust) collection and disposal. For each ingredient or item of waste, thought must be given to:

What is to be collected?

What quantities are expected?

How must the waste be moved through and out of the area to prevent accumulation and possible contamination?

How must the material be disposed off: municipal sewage, landfill or incineration?

Organising for Cleaning

Effective cleaning of both physical facility and equipment is enhanced by facility design details, which reduce bacterial growth areas, minimise contaminant collection points and improve surface cleanability. Beyond design details, broader consideration must be given for the space and utility needs of cleaning.

Cleaning Equipment

Cleaning equipment must be controlled like all other equipment entering controlled environments. It must be cleaned, sanitised and, where necessary, sterilised if for ultra clean use. After use, the equipment must be removed from the controlled area for storage and cleaning prior to reuse. The equipment required will depend on individual needs but may include buckets, mops, sponges, spray guns, brushes and vacuum hoses. Areas must be provided adjacent to the controlled environment where cleaning equipment can be cleaned and stored without subjecting it to potential contamination.

Utility Requirements

Utility needs for aseptic zone cleaning are unique. Both sewage drains and non-aseptic water supplies are contamination potentials to be avoided. Use of Water for Injection or DM/DI filtered water eliminates the potential water contamination. After cleaning, the wastewater may be picked up by mops, which may redistribute contamination rather than remove it. One alternate approach is to spray the cleaning solution onto the surface and remove it by a central vacuum collection system. The vacuum connections are sanitised as part of the area cleaning activity to prevent contamination of the clean environment. Although this method is effective, the vacuum piping must be planned and installed in the walls of the facility during construction.

Cleaning Auxiliary Areas

Auxiliary areas are those places upstream of the controlled environment in which packaging components, and processing equipment are cleaned and sterilised, and in which chemicals are blended into clean bulk formulations.

The ceiling, lighting fixtures (inside and outside), sprinkler heads and air supply vents are thoroughly washed with a microbicidal detergent solution and cloth. Burned-out bulbs are replaced with new ones that have been similarly wiped. Then walls, including baseboards, doors, doorframes and air return vents are thoroughly washed.

Following this, all horizontal surfaces, fixtures, equipment and furniture are washed and wiped. Accessible floor areas and cover bases are vacuumed and machine scrubbed, with a final wipe with clean water.

Cleaning the Critical Zone

The controlled environment in which the critical process is carried out is cleaned using the procedures outlined for auxiliary areas. One significant difference to be borne in mind is that there are no drains provided in a controlled environment, since they are a potential source of contaminants. Liquid spills in controlled environs should be removed with a wet/dry vacuum fitted with a HEPA exhaust, followed by a damp wipe down with microbicidal detergent solution.

Cleaning Service Areas

For purposes of definition, a service area includes offices, rest rooms, storage rooms, mechanical support rooms, lockers and rooms downstream of the controlled processes.

Qualification of Cleaning

- ***Direct surface testing***
    - White light
    - Contaminant Illuminator
    - Optical Microscopy
    - SEM
    - Laser scatter
    - EDXA
    - X-Ray/UV Photoelectron spectroscopy
- ***Anthracine powder test***
- ***Rinse sampling and conductivity tests***
  (check not only for residues but also for potential contaminants)
- ***Identification of soil, residue help determine source***
- ***Caution in sampling***
    - ***Sampling material may interfere with sample***
    - ***Residue may not be soluble or be physically occuded***
    - ***Soil may not be uniformly distributed***

The ceilings are wiped down with a microbicidal detergent solution using a sponge or cloth. The sprinkler heads are dusted with a soft-bristled brush and light diffusers are cleaned using detergent solution. Where drapes are unavoidable, a vacuum cleaner equipped with a brush tool is used. The air supply and return vents are washed with a degreasing microbicidal detergent solution and sponge. A microbicidal detergent solution is used to wipe down the walls, door and partitions. The cloth or sponge employed in such operations must always be of a non-shedding type to reduce particulation. The windows are washed with a suitable window cleaner. Accessible areas of office furniture and other miscellaneous equipment are damp wiped using a microbicidal detergent solution and cloth.

Rest rooms are especially hard to clean and require great care. Sinks and bowls and related plumbing hardware are washed with a microbicidal detergent and cloth. The interior surfaces of all bowls are cleaned with hydrochloric acid.

In mechanical support rooms, lockers and storage rooms, accessible floor areas and cover bases are vacuumed and then machine scrubbed. The floor is then rinsed with clean water. The floor drains and drinking fountain drains are flushed with a microbicidal detergent solution.

Equipment Cleaning

Equipment cleaning, like facility cleaning, requires consideration during planning stages. It lends itself to a central operation, at least for closely allied production areas, but cannot be located in such a way that travel through non-controlled areas is required. Equipment cleaning involves not only the process machinery but also all associated auxiliaries like pumps, hoses, pipes, fittings and filters. The cleaning may involve disassembly, removal of product residue, reassembly, integrity testing, sterilisation and storage. The area should be separate from, but adjacent to the clean production area, and will probably function at irregular hours. An adequate supply of water, including pure water, steam, compressed air, nitrogen, is typically required. If equipment is to be used aseptically, provision must be made for sterilisation prior to use.

Validation of the Cleaning Process

- *Enunciate the objective of validation*
- *Determine number of cleaning processes for a task*
- *Consider both chemical and microbiological contaminants for CIP systems*
- *Examine the detail and specificity of a procedure*
- *Document criticial cleaning steps*
- *Record cleaning, residues after cleaning and variance in test results*
- *Check flow charts and piping diagrams for identification of valves and written cleaning procedures*
- *Determine the specificity and sensitivity of the analytical method for detection of residuals, with special reference to the instrument's LOD*
- *Check manner of setting limits for acceptance*
- *Remember that a procedure that requires repeated retesting is indicative of invalid cleaning process (assumption being that tests are infallible, and samples are representative)*

Preparation, like planning, is a vital part of the manufacturing process. Preparation of equipment entails the cleaning, sanitising, assembling, and in many cases, sterilising and/or depyrogenation of equipment, which may include items as diverse as tanks, mixers, process equipment, transfer lines and the work area in general. The proper cleaning of all equipment that comes in contact with the product is particularly critical. Concern must be demonstrated for general cleanliness as well as for the equipment and area, so that one must be sure that the area and equipment are free from cross-contamination from products processed just previously, or those being processed nearby.

The first step in maintaining clean equipment is the practice of ordinary good housekeeping practices. Orderliness and cleanliness are prerequisites for proper aseptic zone operation. Equipment should never be put away dirty. Cleaning up as soon as possible after an operation has been completed is good practice. Dirty equipment can supply the contaminants, both viable and nonviable, to compromise other portions of the facility. Nothing substitutes for good nonabrasive scrubbing with microbicidal detergent solution followed by wipe down with clean water.

Because some equipment are very complex, chemical tests are often employed to detect residual detergents in the rinse water, and rinsing is continued until the level is below maximum acceptable limits. Where possible, drying should be under LAF cover; and storage must be under lint-free wraps in a clean, dry area.

Microbial purity of water for cleaning should meet PHS standards with not more than 500 CFU/ml. Final rinse is recommended with pure water at a temperature of 80 °C with not more than 100CFU/ml.

Validation of Cleaning

Validation of cleaning procedures has generated considerable discussion since agency documents, including the Inspection Guide for Bulk Drug Substances and the Biotechnology Inspection Guide, briefly addressed this issue. Orange Guide 2002 has included validation of cleaning in its Anexure 15.

Guides are designed to establish inspection consistency and uniformity by discussing practices that have been found to be acceptable, or unacceptable. At the same time one must recognise that for cleaning validation, as with validation of other processes, there may be more than one way to validate a process. In the end, the test of any validated process is whether scientific data shows that the system consistently performs as expected, and produces results that consistently meet predetermined specifications.

The first step is to focus on the objective of the validation process. It is not unusual to see manufacturers use extensive testing and sampling programmes following the cleaning process without ever really evaluating the effectiveness of the steps used to clean the process. Several questions need to be addressed when evaluating the cleaning process. For example, at what point does a piece of equipment or system become *clean*? Does it have to be scrubbed by hand? What is accomplished by hand scrubbing rather than just a solvent wash? How variable are manual cleaning processes from batch to batch, and product to product? How can you be sure you have done the job well if you cannot see the soil before, during or after the operation? The answers to these questions are obviously important to the inspection and evaluation of the cleaning process, since one must evaluate the overall effectiveness of the process. Answers to these questions may also identify steps that can be eliminated for more effective measures and result in resource savings for the company.

Cleaning Validation

- Cleaning validation should be performed in order to confirm the effectiveness of a cleaning procedure. The rationale for selecting limits of carry over of product residues, cleaning agents and microbial contamination should be logically based on the materials involved. The limits should be achievable and verifiable.
- Validated analytical methods having sensitivity to detect residues or contaminants should be used. The detection limit for each analytical method should be sufficiently sensitive to detect the established acceptable level of the residue or contaminant.
- Normally only cleaning procedures for product contact surfaces of the equipment need to be validated. Consideration should be given to non-contact parts. The intervals between use and cleaning as well as cleaning and reuse should be validated. Cleaning intervals and methods should be determined.
- For cleaning procedures for products and processes which are similar, it is considered acceptable to select a representative range of similar products and process. A single validation study utilising a 'worst case' approach can be carried out which takes account of the critical issues.
- Typically three consecutive applications of the cleaning procedure should be performed and shown to be successful in order to prove that the method is validated.
- '*Test until clean*' is not considered an appropriate alternative to cleaning validation.
- Products which simulate the physicochemical properties of the substances to be removed may exceptionally be used instead of the substances themselves, where such substances are either toxic or hazardous.

Determine the number of cleaning processes for pieces of equipment. Ideally, a piece of equipment or system will have one process for cleaning, irrespective of the product or substance being cleaned. However, in some cases, particularly in Research & Development manufacturing areas for clinical products, multiple processes and a variety of solvents may have to be employed.

Examine the design of the equipment, particularly in those large systems that may employ clean-in-place (CIP) or automation, since they represent significant concerns. For example, sanitary type piping without ball valves should be used; if not, the cleaning process may be more difficult. The bulk drug industry utilises non-sanitary ball valves. When such systems are identified, it is important that the operators performing the cleaning operations be aware of problems, and receive special training in cleaning these systems and valves. Determine whether the cleaning operators have adequate knowledge, level of training and experience both of the systems and the cleaning process. Also check the written and validated cleaning process to ascertain if the systems have been properly identified and validated.

Consider both microbiological and chemical contaminants in these CIP systems. You may, for example, find Pseudomonas sp. contamination in a drug substance caused by improper sanitisation of the piping between reactors and the bulk drug manufacturing equipment.

Examine the detail and specificity of the procedure for the cleaning process being validated, and the amount of documentation required. It may be a generic SOP; or a log sheet system requiring some specific documentation for each step. Depending on the complexity of the system and the cleaning process, and the ability and training of the operators, the amount of documentation for executing various cleaning steps or procedures will vary.

When more complex cleaning procedures are required, it is important to document the critical cleaning steps. However, for relatively simple cleaning operations, like machine washing of bags used for dryers, vacuum systems or centrifuges, the mere documentation that the overall cleaning process was performed might suffice.

Other factors such as history of cleaning, residue levels found after cleaning, and variances in test results may also dictate the amount of documentation required. For example, when variable residue levels are detected following cleaning, particularly for a process that is believed to be acceptable, one must establish the effectiveness of the process and operator performance. Appropriate evaluations must be made and when operator performance is deemed a problem, more extensive guidance/documentation and training may be required.

In some of the larger systems, such as those employing long transfer lines or piping, check the flow charts and piping diagrams for the identification of valves and written cleaning procedures. Piping and valves should be tagged and easily identifiable by the operator performing the cleaning function. There are reports of incorrect cleaning practices caused by inadequately identified valves, both on prints and physically. Always check for the presence of an often critical element in the documentation of the cleaning process: identifying and controlling the length of time between the end of processing and each cleaning step. This is especially important if the drying of residues will affect the efficiency of a cleaning process.

Determine the specificity and sensitivity of the analytical method used to detect residual contaminants. With advances in analytical technology, residues from the manufacturing and cleaning processes can be detected at very low levels. It should be borne in mind that if residual contaminants are not detected, it is no guarantee that there are no residuals; it only means that the concentration

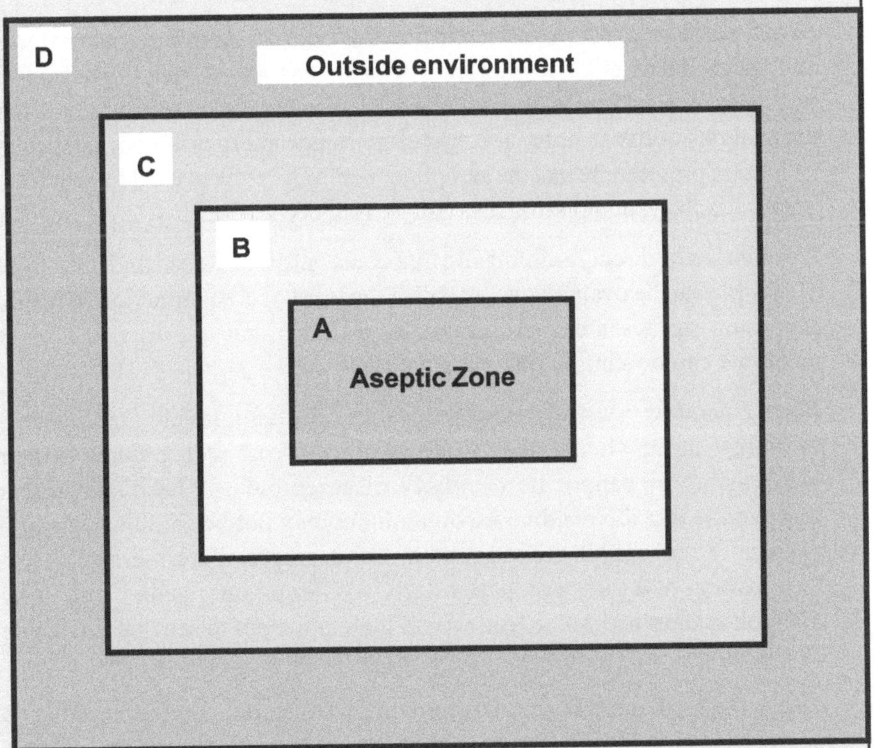

It is recommended practice to first demarcate and grade your controlled environment, so that sanitation stringency increases towards the core locations. This is called *zoning*. On a floor map of the aseptic zone different areas are coloured differently, coded to signify the sanitation stringency prescribed for each. Red is usually reserved for the most critical sites, while green is forbidden, since no area anywhere in or around an aseptic zone can be deemed safe.

Fig.8.1: Zoning the Workplace

of residuals is below the limit of detection (LOD). There are reports of UV scanning of samples with little or no knowledge of the detection limit of the test: at what concentration will the test identify the contaminate.

There are two general types of sampling that have been found acceptable. The most desirable is the direct method of sampling the surface of the object cleaned. A less desirable method is the use of rinse solutions. The use of a pseudo product or placebo is not generally acceptable.

Direct surface sampling: Determine the type of sampling material used and ascertain whether it interferes with or has any other impact on the test data. For example, the adhesive used in swabs often interferes with the analysis of the sample. It is therefore important to establish early in the validation programme that the sampling media and solvent used for extraction are satisfactory, compatible and can be reliably utilised.

Advantages of direct sampling are that areas hardest to clean and reasonably accessible can be evaluated to establish the level of contamination or residue per given surface area. Additionally, residues that are dried out or are insoluble can be sampled by physical removal.

Rinse Samples: Two advantages of using rinse samples are that it enables sampling and evaluation of larger surface areas, and systems that are inaccessible or cannot be routinely disassembled. The disadvantage, however, is that the residue or contaminant may not be soluble, or may be physically occluded in the equipment. For example, if you were evaluating the cleaning of a dirty pot, particularly with dried out residue, you would not look at the rinse water; you would look at the pot to see that it is indeed clean.

Check to see that a direct measurement of the residue or contaminant has been made for the rinse water when it is used to validate the cleaning process. For example, it is not acceptable to simply test rinse water for water quality (does it meet compendial tests), rather than test it for potential contaminates.

Indirect testing, such as conductivity testing, may be of some value for routine monitoring once a cleaning process has been validated. This would be particularly true for manufacturers with reactors, centrifuges, or piping connecting large equipment who rely purely on rinse solution sampling.

***Placebo Product*:** A placebo batch is processed in the equipment under essentially the same operating parameters used for processing the product. A sample of the placebo batch is then tested for residual contamination.

Several significant problems have been reported in using this method to validate a cleaning process.

One cannot assume that the contaminate will be uniformly distributed throughout the system. For example, if the discharge valve or chute of a blender are contaminated, the contaminant would probably not be uniformly disbursed in the placebo; it would most likely be concentrated in the initial discharged portion of the batch. Again, if the contaminant or residue was of a larger particle size, it may not be distributed uniformly.

Some have made the assumption that residual contaminants will be worn off the equipment surface uniformly. This need not hold true.

Finally, the analytical power may be greatly reduced through dilution of the concentrate.

Check the manner in which limits are established. If the cleaning method is evaluated and optimised, and sampling and analytical methods established, a pragmatic approach may be used to set a limit.

The manner in which limits have been set by the industry as a whole has been varied and largely arbitrary. For example, some project levels of contamination based on the concept of uniformity of contaminants throughout a system or piece of equipment. They also assume that the contaminant will be uniformly disbursed in the next substance or product processed through the system or equipment. Some even calculate the dose of diluted contaminant based on the therapeutic dose of the following substance or product. Once the theoretical level of contaminant is determined, a safety or toxicological evaluation is feasible.

While there are some who subscribe to this hypothetical exercise, there are others who do not bother about toxicological calculations at this premature stage. They are more concerned that their cleaning processes are evaluated, optimised and made consistent. Only after this is achieved, do they begin with toxicological and safety assessments.

Testing and retesting until clean is acceptable while validating a process; but not thereafter. Any system that calls for repeated retesting implies that it has been assumed that the tests are infallible, and the samples are representative; by corollary, the procedure is not validated.

A validated system prescribes the time, mode, frequency and number of samples and tests, and sets the acceptance limits. Any deviations in results should be taken as a warning that all is not well, implying that the cleaning was not satisfactory or adequate, and recommence cleaning all over again.

Retesting with more and more samples without recleaning, until results are conveniently in the acceptance range is nothing more than an exercise in self-delusion and could seriously jeopardise your contamination control programme.

Practical Methods: To check for residual particulates, an incandescent mercury bulb is used, with the incident beam of white light striking the surface at an angle. This causes scatter of light by the residual particles. Another method is to use a Black Ray lamp, and this causes fluorescence. Most sub-micronic particulates, specially organic substances, do fluoresce, which makes this a useful method for testing. However, both methods, particularly the latter, can damage eyes, and must be used with care without directly looking into the beam, and restricting viewing to short periods. Anthracine powder is often sprinkled on a test surface, and the cleaning is commenced. At the end of the process, the black ray lamp is used to check for residuals. Anthracine fluoresces remarkably, so that the effectiveness of the cleaning process, and the efficiency of the operator carrying out the cleaning, can be judged.

Quantitative analysis of rinse solutions and surface studies using Optical Microscopy, Scanning Electron Microscopy, Laser scatter studies, Electron Dispersive X-Ray Analysis, X-Ray/ UV Photoelectron spectroscopy can provide information about the likely source of the contaminants. For example, latex would point to gloves; magnesium or zinc would point to talcum powder; sodium or potassium may suggest body salts; and lint is certainly from garments.

Cleaning the Aseptic Zone: A Summary

- It is recommended practice to first demarcate and grade your controlled environment, so that sanitation stringency increases towards the core locations. This is called zoning. On a floor map of the aseptic zone different areas are coloured differently, coded to signify the sanitation stringency prescribed for each. Red is usually reserved for the most critical sites, while green is forbidden, since no area anywhere in or around an aseptic zone can be deemed safe.
- Check that all cleaning agents and implements are aseptic zone grade: cleanable, sterilisable and non-contaminating. It is also important to evaluate some other key parameters and characteristics like surface tension, polarity and pH; their solubility, stability and reactivity, including corrosiveness; their efficiency as surfactants; their propensity to leave residues; and most importantly, the recommended use dilution and temperature.
- Prepare a fresh cleaning solution, accurately diluted for each task. Make up only the quantity required in a clean, dry container. Freshly drawn tap water is usually suitable for peripheral areas. Very hard water will precipitate soaps and neutralise some disinfectants. For aseptic processing zones use WFI grade water. Hot water cleans better than cold. But at temperatures above 65 °C it coagulates proteins, and organic stains, if any, will then be more difficult to remove.
- Use of two buckets mounted firmly on a trolley, one for fresh solution and the other for rinsing is common practice; use of three buckets, one marked dirty where the soiled solution is drained, a second marked rinse and last marked clean would be an even more effective procedure.

- Brushes, mops and wipes should be dry and clean before use. Apply the cleaning solution evenly to all of the surfaces. Do not apply more fluid than necessary onto a surface. This avoids waste, seepage into cracks, shrinkage of surface materials, and difficulties of subsequent removal.
- Always clean down from ceiling, walls to floor, from the farthest point to nearest, with gentle, steady, unidirectional strokes. This holds for both wet as well as dry wiping, where the stroke length should not be more than 400 mm. (When dry wiping, expose a fresh, clean surface for each stroke).
- Rinse off cleaning solutions when practical, and change contents frequently to prevent buildup of soil in the solution, which will lead to recontamination.
- Allow sufficient time for cleaning solutions to penetrate the soil on the surface. However, do bear in mind that strong acid or alkaline cleaning agents can damage surfaces if left in contact too long.
- Dispose off used cleaning solution in the manner prescribed by your SOP in the designated area. Do not empty into wash basins or work area sinks.
- Remove any fluid trapped in channels or elsewhere, and dry the cleaned surface as thoroughly as possible.
- Remove cleaning equipment, accessories and implements from the aseptic zone as soon as the cleaning process is completed. Clean them as per methods laid down in your SOP, dry them and store them in the designated location. If the equipment is faulty, report it promptly to your supervisor.
- Wash hands before carrying out any other duties.

9 Sterilisation

Those of you for whom sterilisation is not a nightmare can count your blessings and quietly skip this section, and for good measure, the next and appendix too. But others must bear with both. Though there is little said here that is new, an attempt is made to review the topic in its totality, placing emphasis on aspects that critically influence integrated microcontamination control.

Sterilisation literally implies destruction or elimination of all forms of microbial life. In practice, however, such a state is seldom attained, because of the temporal characteristics of microbial resistance. It is recognised that inactivation of microorganisms is a time-dependent process, influenced by initial microbial population, rate and duration of biocidal action. When a homogeneous population of microorganisms is exposed to a lethal agent, only a fixed proportion of the initial population, not the entire population, is deemed to be inactivated per unit of exposure. The number of surviving microorganisms decreases exponentially with time, and the lethality of action, independent of the initial number, until the residual population is below level of detection. This entails establishment of probabilistic rather than absolute criteria for measuring effectiveness of the sterilisation process.

If the initial bioburden on an item is N_0, at a constant lethality factor, the population decreases exponentially to N_t after an interval of time = t. If this ratio is, say, 10^{-6}, it implies that the probability that a microorganism has survived the sterilisation process is one in a million. As a corollary it can be said that if a million such items with identical initial bioburden were subject to the same sterilisation process, you can expect to find one that remains unsterile.

This estimation of Probability of Survivor per Item (PSI) led to the acceptance of Sterility Assurance Level (SAL), of a prescribed limit as an adequate guarantee that the sterilisation process has been satisfactory. For example, according to current compendial standards, for a pharmaceutical product or a medical device to be labeled sterile, it is generally considered that on completion of the sterilisation process, the theoretical probability of there being one viable microorganism shall be equal to or less than one in a million processed items, and is referred to as an SAL equal to or better than 10^{-6}.

The core problem in any sterilisation process is the attainment of the recommended SAL without any compromise in product integrity and functionality. Since the product with its initial bioburden is an integral unit, the sterilisation process must be prospectively designed into the product. Extensive research on sterilisation has resulted in a great deal of detailed information on the death of microorganisms. There are difficulties in defining death. Death cannot be defined by positive criteria; it can be characterised only by the absence of some property which is essential to life.

The different criteria of death refer to the inactivation of different mechanisms which are indispensable for the life and reproduction of the cell. These mechanisms can be divided into five groups, according to the function they control:

Group I : Mechanisms controlling the passage of substances into and out of the cell represented by the cell membrane.

Group II : Mechanisms controlling the energy production for all life activity, comprising enzymes.

Group III : Mechanisms which probably involve a large number of different catalysts that control the synthesis of the cell constituents.

Group IV : Mechanisms controlling multiplication known to have their seat in the nuclei in higher organisms.

Group V : Mechanisms consisting of protein molecules which often make up the bulk of the cytoplasm, such as myosin, leguminium, glutinin, and the globulins of bacterin. These are without definitely known physiological functions, but are essential for the life of the cell since their denaturation causes death.

Spore death is generally believed to be the result of an irreversible denaturation of protein and nucleic acids, brought about by the cleavage of critical hydrogen bonds resulting in permanent alteration of tertiary peptide and polynucleotide structures. Since it is the same biochemical structures in any strain, specific population of spores that undergo denaturation, the efficacy of the method for inactivating these spores should not vary to any great extent when inoculated into various formulations. Though this premise is largely supported, the rate constants differ by a factor of 20, reflecting the effectiveness of formulation variables in penetration of the inactivating agent which causes denaturation through the spore coat and cortex. One such variable is acidity, which is recognised to encourage speedy transfer of hydrogen ions through the spore coat and cortex, causing spore death. Acidic conditions in synergistic combination with the inactivating agent result in rapid spore death.

Precise mathematical expressions have been derived to characterise microbial inactivation patterns, and identify elements that influence the process. For example holding time (duration of exposure of the product to the lethal agent) and the inactivation parameter (temperature in heat sterilisation, dosage level in radiation, concentration of chemical in disinfection, filter efficiency in membrane sterilisation) help determine the efficiency of the sterilisation process.

At this stage it helps to refresh our memory with the mathematical expressions of microbial resistance that play a part in the development of sterilisation procedures.

The achievement of sterility within any one item in a population of items submitted to a sterilisation process can neither be guaranteed nor demonstrated. The inactivation of microorganisms by physical or chemical means follows an exponential law, asymptotically approaching zero, and governed by the formula :

$N = N_0 \, e^{-kt}$ where

N_0 = Initial bioburden

N = Residual bioburden

k = "kill" rate of the inactivation method used

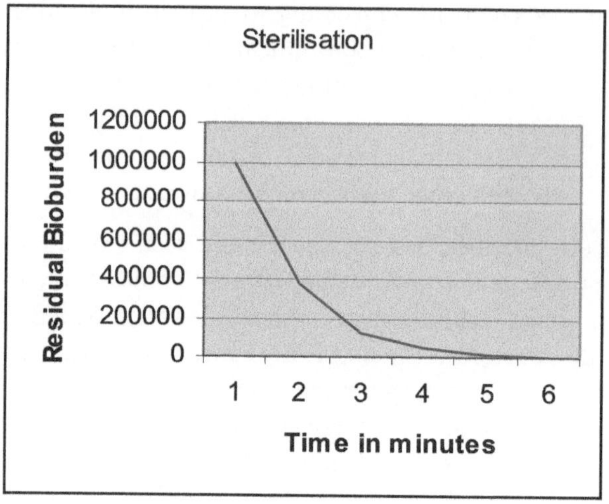

Fig.9.1: Bioburden decay

t = time subjected to inactivation agent

Using logarithm to the base 10, the same equation may be written as

$$N = N_0 10^{-k\,t/2.3} \text{ or}$$
$$\log (N / N_0) = -k\,t / 2.3 \text{ or}$$
$$\log (N_0 / N) = k\,t / 2.3$$

The ratio (N_0 / N) is referred to as

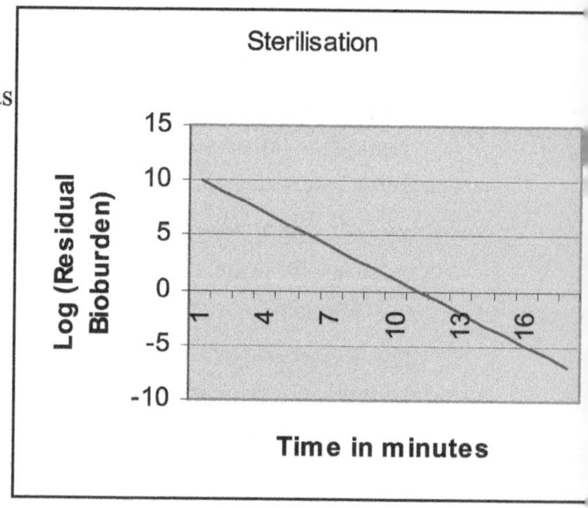

Fig.9.2: Bioburden decay on log scale

The curve dips below the X-axis, and the corresponding readings on the Y-axis are negative. For example, a residual bioburden of 10^{-3} means that 1 in every 1000 is still alive; 10^{-6} means one in every million survives.

Thus there is always a finite statistical probability that a microorganism may survive the sterilisation process. This is called the Probability of Survivor Index **(PSI)**.

For a given process, the PSI is determined by the number, types and resistance of the microorganisms present and by the environment in which the organisms exist during treatment.

The sterility assurance limit **(SAL)** of a sterilising process is the degree of assurance with which the process in question renders a population of items sterile. The SAL for a given process is expressed as the probability of a non-sterile item in that population. An SAL of 10^{-6}, for example, denotes a probability of not more than one viable microorganism in 1×10^{6} sterilised items of the final product. If the initial bioburden is 10^{8}, and after the inactivation treatment it is reduced to 10, the total "log reduction" is by a factor of 8 as shown below:

$$\log (N_0/N) = \log (IF) = \log (10^{8}/10) = 8$$

If our initial bioburden is 10^{4} and we want this reduced to an SAL of 10^{-6} we need a tenfold reduction in the log value

$$\log (IF) = \log (N_0/N) = \log (10^{4} / 10^{-6}) = 10$$

The time required to bring about a reduction in log value by one (or one decimal value reduction in the initial bioburden, or inactivate or destroy 90% of the initial viable microbial population) is called the D-value.

D-value suffix refers to inactivating agent's level/rate. For example, in moist steam method, the D-value at T = 121°C is referred to as D_{121}

Inactivation rate may refer to just one parameter like dosage level or temperature, or a combination of parameters like temperature, pressure, pH etc.

Simple mathematics shows that the equation for the inactivation factor may be re-written in terms of the Decimal-reduction value as:

$$IF = (N_0/N) = 10^{t/D}$$

During the sterilisation process, the inactivating agent delivers lethality *over the period of treatment.* In the case of heat sterilisation, heat is delivered during the heating up, holding and cooling down phases of the cycle. The sum total of full lethal dose, from start of cycle to finish takes, let us say, F minutes to deliver, and bring the bioburden down to the desired SAL of 10^{-6}. Then this process of inactivation can be represented by

$$IF = (N_0/N) = 10^{F/D}$$

In the case of saturated steam sterilisation, for example, the total cycle

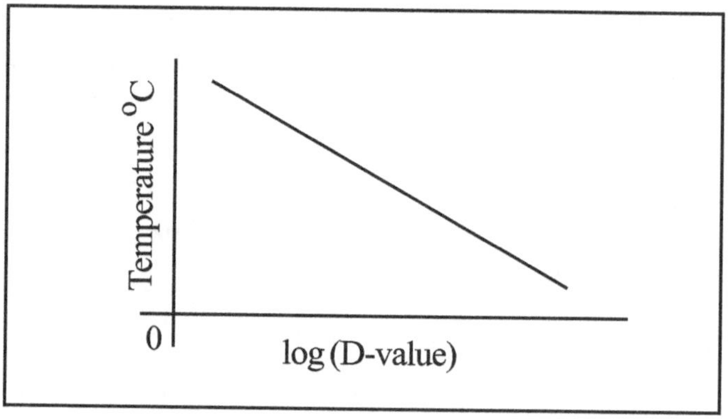

Fig.9.3

time required at a temperature of 121 °C for achieving the desired inactivation level is referred to as F_o (F sub-zero), and the process is represented as:

$$\log (IF) = \log (N_0/N) = F_o / D_{121} \text{ or}$$

$$F_o = D_{121} \log (IF)$$

As we raise the temperature in heat sterilisation the time to bring down the bioburden by 90% or one log-scale reduction reduces progressively. In other words, as temperature rises, the corresponding D-value falls. If we were to plot Temperature against the logarithm of the D-value we find the relationship is linear.

$$T_2 - T_1 = -z \log (D_2 / D_1) = z \log (D_1 / D_2)$$

If $\log (D_1 / D_2) = 1$, then

$$Z = T_2 - T_1$$

The rise in temperature to bring about a one log-scale reduction in the D-value (reduce to one-tenth of the original value) is referred to as the **z-value**.

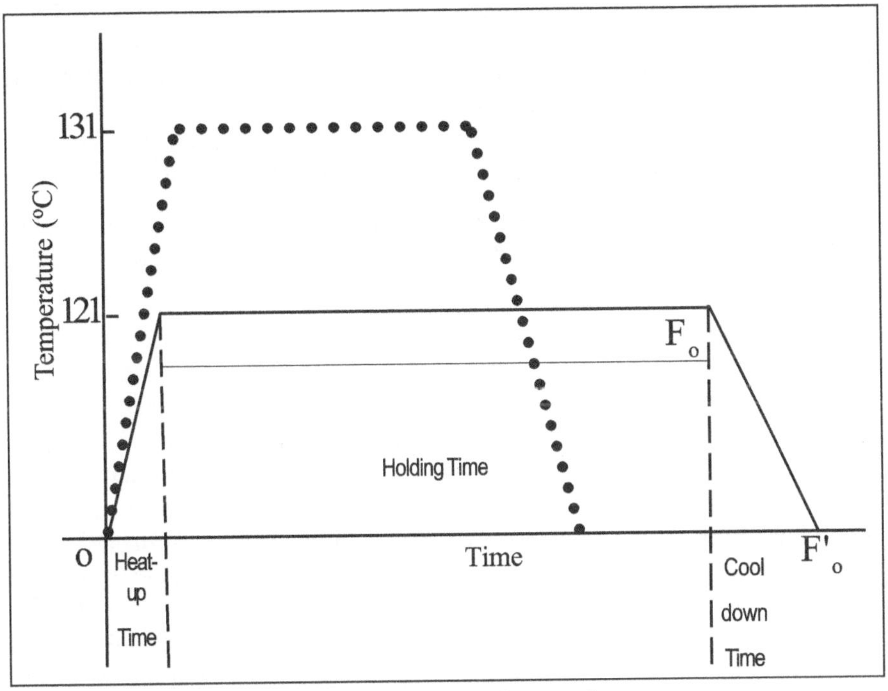

Fig.9.4: Sterilisation cycle

In heat sterilisation, z-value is constant over temperature ranges. The mean value in moist heat sterilisation (*B. stearothermophilus*) is 10°C, and for dry heat sterilisation (*B.subtilis*) is 22°C.

The F-value decreases with D-value. Since D-value reduces with increase in Temperature, it effectively means that a sterilisation cycle time can be reduced to achieve the same SAL. In addition to temperature levels, rate of change of temperature also influences the inactivation efficacy and time.

This gives us an excellent opportunity to explore ways and means of reducing the time and resources consumed by the sterilisation process.

The area under the curve represents the sum total of lethal heat energy delivered. In the above figure, two curves are shown; if the area under each is the same, it implies that the same amount of lethal heat energy has been delivered. The curve indicated with dotted lines represents a sterilisation cycle that has been completed in less time than the process represented by solid lines. Once the former cycle is validated, the User has benefited by the time he has saved.

In developing a sterilisation process the number and range of the variables influencing the process must be determined and their interaction with the product must be studied, especially to check that there are no deleterious effects. This involves ascertaining the product susceptibility parameters to the lethal agent employed. Preservation of product quality, chemical purity, potency and functionality are prime considerations. Testing is also required to determine the maximum rate of change in the parameters (pressure, concentration, pH or temperature) tolerated by the product and packaging.

Three recognised process approaches are used to design a sterilisation process: Overkill, absolute bioburden and a combination of biological indicator with bioburden.

The overkill approach is employed where the primary concern is assurance of stability and not product degradation. This is possible if it is already known that the product is not adversely affected by the sterilisation process selected. The design aims to inactivate a microbial challenge that is greater in number and resistance than the natural bioburden associated with the product. Moist heat sterilisation, for example, uses B. stearothermophilus whose D-, z- values are considerably higher than those of typical microbial isolates from production environments. *The F-value relating to such a reference organism is referred to as the F_0 of the sterilisation process selected.* When the overkill method is used, there is little need to conduct bioburden studies. Nevertheless, it is good manufacturing practice to carry out periodic microbial audits to ensure that no unusual heat resistant organism is present.

But remember that B. stearothermophilus is unlikely to be around in your production environment, and by using it as the reference you are probably consuming excessive time and resources. Especially if product stability is likely to be endangered, the bioburden approach should be preferred, where individual product bioburden isolates are cultured and harvested and their resistance to the lethal agent determined. The isolate with the highest resistance is used to challenge the process in numbers greater than or equal to the maximum product bioburden.

Another approach is to determine the mean product bioburden level and add three standard deviations (the 6-sigma technique in statistics) to assure an adequate challenge. The process time required to bring down the initial product bioburden to log 10^0 is first determined, and then extended sufficiently to attain a further log scale reduction of 6 to guarantee SAL of 10^{-6} for the product.

The absolute bioburden approach requires extensive ongoing monitoring to screen and check the resistance of isolates at each manufacturing site since specific product bioburdens may differ. A major cause for worry with this approach is that the process of culturing the isolates may change their resistance. Since the most resistant isolate is used as the challenge, the vigil for detecting isolates with higher resistance must continue as an ongoing exercise. The cost of such nonstop screening programme must be weighed against the savings in energy and time that accrue while deciding on this sterilisation approach.

An acceptable compromise is adopting the combination of a biological indicator (BI) with the product bioburden. This requires complete information about the enumeration and resistance of the latter, so that a meaningful relationship may be established with the former. If the product related bioburden is controlled at a lower population level, more resistant bioburden can be tolerated in the defined sterilisation cycle, resulting in much shorter process time than overkill methods.

The different methods of sterilisation in common use today are briefly described here. Whichever method is employed, the points we have made about intelligent use of D-, z- and F- values, and criteria for choice of overkill, bioburden or BI approach apply equally.

Ultraviolet (UV) radiation is used primarily for treating air, large fixed surfaces and water. UV radiation has poor penetrating power, specially in water. Recommended wavelength is in the range of 250-280 nm and radiation level is 3 mw/sq cm. Its mode of action is through blockage of DNA replication by cross-linkage of pyridine bases. They are useful as bacteriostatic agents, but require long exposure periods to be effective. The effectiveness decreases with use and distance of surface from tube. Replacement is advised after of 600 hrs of use or when the intensity level falls to 60% of its original value. It must be borne in mind that the wavelength increases with ageing, and as it approaches 360 nm it progressively turns from a lethal agent into a repellant and on to an attractant.

Irradiation disrupts DNA and RNA in living organisms, and is used by hospital and laboratory suppliers for materials that do not tolerate heat and pressure (i.e., autoclaving) or chemical treatments. It is an applicable decontaminating agent for materials that are thermolabile and/or whose end use does not allow for chemical residue contamination. Before deciding on this option careful evaluation of the effects of this process on the physicochemical properties of all components is recommended.

Ionisation or Gamma emitting Cobalt-60 and Cesium-137 and electron beams are especially useful for materials that are thermolabile and moisture-labile. Mode of action is through Beta radiation that directly damages DNA and denatures proteins. Indirectly it may also generate free radicals from menstruum that may have antimicrobial activities. This method has high penetrating power, but the setup is complicated, expensive and requires a high level of safety precautions.

Infrared radiation: used for heat treatment of small metal and glass items.

Microwaves: used for treatment of liquids, nonmetallic objects, and biohazardous waste.

Membrane filtration physically removes particulates (e.g., microorganisms) from heat-sensitive pharmaceutical and biological fluids. The size of the particles removed is determined by the pore size of the filter membrane is excellent for applications involving liquids and gases, and this method has gained in popularity because of its simplicity, ease in use and validation.

Heat is universally regarded as the most reliable, versatile method of sterilisation. Heat is a non-quantised form of energy and therefore its lethal effect on cells is more likely to be due to an accumulation of irreparable damage resulting from generalised chemical reactions within the cell, than destruction of a specific target molecule. The lethal chemical actions occur more readily in the hydrated state than in the dry state, which is why moist heat is the preferred form of thermal sterilisation for items that are not thermolabile or moisture sensitive.

Dry heat and steam represent the two limits of water vapour concentration. Dry heat sterilisation conditions can be characterised by relative humidity (rh) or water activity (A_w) of 0; whereas steam corresponds to rh of 100% or A_w of 1. Varying conditions exist between these states.

The precise effect of moisture on the lethal rate is due to the fact that spores are highly permeable and free exchange of water occurs between the spore and its environment. This exchange varies with changes in the rh of the environment. Content and location of water in spores and dehydration of spore protoplast are the predominant physicochemical factors affecting spore resistance to moist heat. Detailed studies on effects in moist heat processes.

The enhanced kill rate in moist heat processes is also evident in the differences in temperature required for moist heat vs dry heat. Typically dry heat processes are run at 160 °C or higher, whereas moist heat temperatures vary from 115 °C to 135 ^{0}C. This is due to the fact that steam contains high latent heat, whereas air has low latent heat.

Since moist heat sterilisation requires ready access to steam or hot water source, it is confined to batch treatment; in contrast the relative ease with which air can be heated lends dry heat sterilisation convenient for continuous on-line treatment.

Moist heat has different forms: dry saturated steam, superheated steam, wet steam, steam-air mixes, and superheated water spray or water immersion. Dry saturated steam is most efficacious in its sterilising effects as it provides the optimum combination of heat content, moisture content and penetrability required for biocidal action.

Chemical sterilisation, commonly referred to as disinfection, is regarded as an option to be avoided, if possible, mainly because it is a foreign substance that must come in contact with the product or contact parts before it can act; it may leave residues; it may not be easy to clean off after use, and because the action is often uncertain and difficult to monitor, repeat or sustain. Besides, unlike other modes of sterilisation, chemical disinfection is generally believed to inactivate vegetative bacteria and lipid viruses, with variable, perhaps even doubtful, effect on spores and other forms of microbial flora. But more about this in the next chapter.

Some of the methods for sterilisation described may be applied in combination to produce enhanced or synergistic activity. Combination of some chemical agents and heat demonstrate sporicidal activity not exhibited by either agent individually. Ultrasound has been reported to enhance the activity of some chemical agents.

Before we pass on to the criteria for selection of the lethal agents and the sterilising processes, let us pause to consider the wide range and composition of surfaces routinely encountered in cleanrooms. The shell materials include ceramic with vinyl epoxy spray-on, epoxy paint over sheet rock, masonry, glass, PVC, metal panels, walls, ceiling, vinyl sheeting, ceramic-plastic cement tile, and epoxy aggregates or stone tiles for floors. Lighting fixtures feature baked enamel over metal and acrylic plastic. Materials used for plumbing (sinks and floor drains) include stainless steel, brass, PVC and enamel. HVAC ducts are usually constructed of aluminium, stainless steel, galvanised steel or epoxy coated GI. Equipment and materials used in production are typically fabricated from stainless steel, glass, rubber and plastics. Garments worn by personnel to protect against product contamination are usually made from synthetic fibres such as Dacron, Nomex, Nylon, Polyester, Tyvek, treated paper and rubber.

The process of selecting an appropriate decontaminating agent necessitates the consideration of numerous requirements. Various attributes of the surface to be treated (i.e. size and configuration, surface finish, cleanliness, stainability, temperature durability, and wetability), and of the prospective agents should be identified The following questions arise:

- Is the agent effective against the bioburden it will encounter?
- Can the agent be used safely (toxicity, volatility) and economically on the surface to be treated?
- Does the surface shape allow exposure of all critical surfaces to the treatment?
- If the surface is porous, grainy or fibrous, will the agent penetrate all exposed surfaces?
- Must the surface be washed prior to decontamination to remove films or layers of soil that may have been deposited on the surface from a previous operation? Films or soil may interfere with the penetration of the agent to the surface or inactivate the agent.
- Will the surface be altered by the agent (i.e.iodine compounds and glutaraldehyde stain, chlorine compounds bleach, alcohols cause plastics to cloud)?
- Can the surface be heat treated?
- Will moisture interfere with the use or function of the surface?
- If an agent such as an aldehyde, phenolic, halaphore, quat or ethylene oxide (EtO) is used, will the residue deposited on the treated surface potentiate product contamination?
- Will the agent corrode or destroy the treated surface? Iodophors, chlorine compounds and peroxides are generally corrosive. (Glutaraldehyde corrodes carbon steel; steam dulls sharp edges.)
- Will the method of preparation or application of an agent influence its activity or effectiveness? The activity of some chemical agents is affected by a specific pH, temperature and/or ionic strength of solution.

Table 9.1: Typical Conditions Employed in Sterilisation

Sterilisation method	Conditions
Moist heat (autoclave)	15 psi, 121°C for 15 min 15 psi, 134°C for 3 min
Dry Heat	160°C for 120 min 170°C for 60 min 180°C for 30 min
Ethylene oxide	Gas concentration 800 - 1200 mg/litre 45°C - 63°C 30 - 70% Rh 1 - 4 hours
Low temperature steam and formaldehyde	Gas concentration 15 - 100 mg/litre Steam admission to 73°C 40 - 180 min depending on process
Irradiation	25 kGy (2.5 Mrad) dose Gamma rays or accelerated electrons
Filtration	< 0.22 micron pore size sterile membrane filter

Table 9.2: Sterilisation Process Monitoring

Types of Monitors

1. Electro-mechanical : Pressure, Temperature, Time etc.. (Recommend Automation)

2. Chemical : Fusible pellet in sealed glass tube: melts, color changes
Temperature sensitive coloured solution - Browne's tube
Temperature sensitive chemical - Wax melts & exposes mark
Thermochromic chemical - ink undergoes colour change

Biological Indicators

1 Paper carrier Biological Indicators
2 Self-contained Biological Indicators - Ampoules
3 Spore suspensions

Sterilizalion Process	Species	Inoculam size	D-value
Autoclave (121°C)	Bacillus stearothermophilus	> 10^5	1.5 min
	Clostridium sporogenes	> 10^8	0.8 min
Dry heat (160°C)	Bacillus subtilis var. niger	> 10^5	5 - 10 min
Ethylene Oxide	Bacillus subtilis var. niger	10^6 - 10^7	9 min.
Ionization radiation	Bacillus pumilus	10^7 - 10^8	3kGy (022) (0.3 Mrad)
Filtration (0.22m)	Ps.Diminuta	depends on challenge conditions	

Table 9.3: Heat Sterilization: a comaparative study

	Principle/ Conditions	Advantages	Disadvantages	Uses
Dry Heat	Thermal in activation: destroys by oxidation	Non-corrosive simple design and principle	Less effective than moist heat; requires longer times and/or higher temperatures	Materials that are damaged by, or are impenetrable to, moist heat
Hot Air Oven	160-180ºC for 2-4 hours	Penetrates water-insoluble materials (e.g., grease and oil) less corrosive to metals and sharp instruments than steam	Slow diffusion, penetration loading, packing critical to performance not suitable for reusable plastics	Anhydrous materials, such as oils, greases and powders laboratory glssware, instruments closed containers
Red-heat Flame	Oxidation to ashes (burning)	Rapid	Initial contact with flame can produce a viable aerosol possibility of accidental fire	Inoculating loops, needles
Incineration	Oxidation to ashes (burning) 1-60 minutes: temperatures may exceed 1000ºC	Reduces volume of waste by up to 95%	Improper use may lead to emission of pethogens in smoke requires transport of infectious waste excess plastic (>20%) content reduces combustibility	For decontamination of waste items prior to disposal in landfill
Moist Heat	Irreversible coagulation of (micro bial) proteins	More rapid and more effective than dry heat		
Pasteurization	Heating to below boiling point (generally 77ºC) for up to 30 minutes	Can be used on heat sensitive liquids and medical devices low cost	Not reliably sporicidal	Milk and dairy products some heat - sensitive medical equipment
Tyndallization (Fractional Sterilization)	Heating to 80-100ºC for 30 mins on successive days, with incubation periods in between.	Resistant spores germinate and are killed on the second and third days	Time consuming not reliably sporicidal	Heat sensitive materials such as bacteriologic media, solutions of chemicals, biological materials
Boiling	Maximum temperature obtainable is approximately 100ºC 10-30 mins	Minimal equiment required	Cumbersome: not practical for every day lab use not reliably sporicidal	Small instruments and equipment
Autoclaving	Steam under pressure 121ºC/15 psi for 15-90 mins	Minimal time required most dependable	Loading and packing critical to performance	Penetration of sterile glss ware, media and instruments

10 Good Disinfection Practice

Present practice is far from satisfactory in the use of disinfectants. Every institution often has a different disinfection programme, and the choice of disinfectants for similar purposes varies considerably. A wide range of disinfectants is used, some of which are clearly unsuited for the purpose for which they are employed. In dispensing solutions, members of staff apparently rely upon such measures as a *tablespoonful to a bucket, until it looks enough* and *depending on the smell.* The important principle of *strong enough for long enough* is generally overlooked. Too often, their abuse leads to a dangerous notion of security.

Antiseptics, Disinfectants and Germicides

Terms like antiseptics, disinfectants and germicides are often used interchangeably without drawing distinctions. While all three have antimicrobial action, antiseptics are intended for clinical use, while disinfectants are for use on inanimate objects. The term *germicide* is all embracing to mean fungicide, bactericide, sporicide and viricide. As mentioned earlier, though some chemical agents are effective against all varieties of microbial flora, there is a general tendency to dismiss disinfectants as being useful only against vegetative bacteria and lipid viruses.

Planned Disinfection

Floor cleaning mops, wipes, baths, bath mops and brushes, wash bowls, nail brushes and communal jars containing antiseptics and soap are confirmed sources of contamination and microbes. Antimicrobial chemicals must be properly applied if they are to be of service. Each facility should adopt a properly planned programme on the kind and concentrations of disinfectants to be used for particular purposes, a system of supervision to ensure that the staff are implementing this programme and a system of in-use tests to be made on samples of the disinfectant solutions actually being used in the different areas to ascertain and confirm that they are at the correct concentration and retain adequate activity.

Application Methods

Disinfectants may be applied using a variety of methods, as dictated by their nature and the surface to be treated. Agents prepared as liquids may be applied by:

Spraying is convenient for small to medium size surfaces. However, diluted agents should not be stored in a spray bottle for long periods of time. Time of storage is dependent upon the chemical stability of the agent and the potential for the applicator to become a reservoir for resistant organisms.

Wiping is effective for small to medium size surfaces. Wiping combines the chemical activity of the agent and the physical removal of organisms or soil by abrasion. Wipes should be clean and non-particulating.

Mopping is appropriate for large environmental surfaces and is accomplished by one of three techniques:

Damp mopping: A clean mop of suitable design is dipped into the agent and squeezed out. The mopped surface remains wet for some time.

Wet mopping: Two buckets of decontaminating solution are prepared according to labeled instructions. A liberal amount of solution from one bucket is applied to the surface; and the mop is then rinsed and squeezed out in the second bucket.

Flood and vacuum: A liberal amount of disinfectant solution is applied to the surface, and after a prescribed time of contact the excess is wet vacuumed from the surface.

Submersion in solutions of chemical agents may be effective for decontaminating small surfaces or equipment. Surface cleanliness is a significant parameter in the effectiveness of this method. The activity of some agents like glutaraldehyde are enhanced when used thus in ultrasonic baths.

Fogging is used for disinfecting rooms and their contents. A solution of an appropriate agent is aerosolised in mist form using a revolving dispenser or other suitable device.. The success of this procedure depends upon covering all surfaces with a fine layer of solution. This success could later translate into a problem if there are insoluble residues, or the film stubbornly adheres to the surface making thorough cleaning difficult.

Fumigation where the chemical agent is applied in a gaseous state, concentrated in enclosed areas either at ambient pressure or under vacuum pressure.

Selection of Agents

For daily routine disinfection selection should favour those that are convenient, safe and non-noxious. The more potent, noxious or toxic agents should be reserved for use on a less frequent basis (weekly or monthly) or when advised due to an increase in the baseline microbial level, presence of unique (i.e. sporeformers) or pathogenic microorganisms, or occurrence of atypical operational circumstances. Use of different types of disinfectants on a rotational basis is practised by many companies. Though theoretically rotating different types of agents prevents buildup of organisms resistant to any one agent, there are pitfalls to be avoided, because not all disinfectants are compatible with one another.

Cost is a relevant factor when choosing disinfectants. Those designed for special purposes may be both unsuitable and too expensive for use as general environmental disinfectants. To be used safely on human tissue a disinfectant would have to be non-toxic, non-allergenic, non-corrosive and have a neutral pH. These properties are expensive to achieve and are usually obtained at the expense of other desirable properties like range of action.

Characteristics of Common Disinfectants

Clear soluble phenolics (*Sudol, Izal. Stericol, Clearsol, Hycolin, Jeye's*) are widely used for disinfection of the inanimate environment and objects, and are active against fungi and bacteria, but not against spores and viruses. Phenols denature cell proteins and enzymes. Use concentration is 1% to 2 %.

They are unsuitable for use on living tissues or any item brought into contact with tissues, unless thoroughly rinsed. Phenols attack rubber and metals. In dilute form they are mildly toxic and mildly irritating. At high concentrations and temperatures, and in acid pH, they are aggressively corrosive and toxic. Damage to surfaces may be caused by prolonged or repeated exposures, specially at high concentrations. Phenolics are not recommended for product contact or storage surfaces.

On the other hand, clear soluble phenolics are relatively cheap, usually stable at use dilutions and are not readily neutralised by organic materials or hard water. Though inactivated by cationic detergents, they are soluble and stable in long chain fatty acid soaps, where they assist in spread and aid cleaning. Pine oil is a popular additive, not only because it improves activity, but also because of the agreeable fragrance.

Hypochlorites (*Chloros, Domestos, Sterite, Parazone, Eusol, Milton, Laktone*) are oxidising agents that are most effective in alkaline pH. They are used for disinfecting the environment, sinks and baths, where bleaching is desirable, and where the strong smell of phenol is not acceptable.

Hypochlorites in buffered solutions of 7.5 pH are active against fungi, bacteria, and spores; at high concentrations they are active even against viruses. Although they can be used for disinfection of product contact and storage surfaces at concentrations as low as 200 ppm of available chlorine they are easily neutralised by proteins at this dilution. Use concentration varies from 10 to 200 ppm of available chlorine. Hypochlorites are inactivated by organic matter and cationic detergents. They react with acids to release chlorine, which can be dangerous. They corrode metal, bleach or damage fabrics, attack plastics and rubber. They are relatively unstable, and have low shelf-life.

Glutaraldehyde (*Cidex*) is commonly used for heat sensitive items. It is stable in acid pH, but more active in alkaline pH, aqueous solution buffered to pH 7.5 to 8.5 with sodium bicarbonate. Items exposed to glutaraldehyde under three hours must be deemed disinfected, not sterilised. The recommended exposure time for full effect is 10 hours. Glutaraldehyde is expensive, unpleasant to handle, corrosive, and toxic. It is compatible with soaps and detergents, but leaves a yellow stain. Despite claims about its stability it is prudent to presume that it is most effective only when used immediately. Most Users apply glutaraldehyde on a weekly basis, rather than continuously. Solutions should be discarded when they become visibly cloudy at any time. Ideally, only an unused solution should be used each time, but the cost may prove prohibitive. The number of uses allowable for a solution must depend on circumstances and an indication of the strength of a solution would be useful.

Iodophors (*Betadine, Servocid, Polysan*) have many properties similar to hypochlorites, including their oxidising action. They are less commonly used for environmental disinfection, but more often used as a skin disinfectant. Iodophors consist of Iodine and a solubiliser, and are relatively nontoxic and may be used in catering hygiene. They are stable over long periods, but should be used immediately once diluted. They possess good penetration properties. They can be washed from fabrics more readily than Iodine. The depth of the colour is related to activity and this may be used as an indicator, although this relationship is not entirely reliable. Iodophors are more expensive than hypochlorites, and allergy is less likely than with Iodine. Concentrated solutions can corrode metals and attack plastics and fabrics.

Quarternary Ammonium Compounds have been evolved as the antiseptics of choice for clinical use that combine microbicidal action with low toxicity and allergenicity. The cost is high; the range is limited. QACs are easily inactivated by anionic soap, and are generally not recommended for disinfection of inanimate objects, unless their low toxicity or compatibility with human tissue are of major importance. Their mode of action is through denaturing cellular proteins and enzymes.

Chlorhexidine (*Hibitane, Hibiscrub*) is a diguanide and a sophisticated and relatively expensive antiseptic. It is more active against gram-negative *cocci* and less against gram-negative *rods*. Sporicidal activity is not significant; virucidal activity is poor. Cetrimide in combination with chlorhexidine (*Savlon*) has an inherent detergent property which makes it useful to clean dirty surfaces. Benzalkonium chloride in aqueous solution with detergents is stable over long periods of time. It is inactivated by anionic soaps, proteins, organic matter and cork under bottle caps, but not by hard water. It is an irritant and can harm the eyes.

Chlorxylenol (*Dettol, Iteol*) is active against fungi and gram-positive cocci, but generally weak against others. It is inactivated by hard water, cork, proteins and organic matter. It is nontoxic and non-irritant, and its activity is enhanced by the chelating action of EDTA.

Alcohol (*Ethanol, Isopropanol*) acts rapidly but penetrates poorly. It is effective mainly against vegetative bacteria and is commonly used for disinfection of clean surfaces, human or inanimate. Its chief advantage is in its quick evaporation, leaving the surface dry almost immediately after use.

The dehydrating effects of alcohol at high concentrations causes problems. Recommended additives are glycerol, chlorhexidine, iodine and in rare cases involving spilled cultures, formaldehyde. Alcohol is inactivated by proteins and organic matter, incompatible with plastics and asphalt, and promote rusting of ferrous materials. It is flammable and requires care in storage and handling.

Hydrogen Peroxide requires protective gear, is toxic, irritant, corrosive and attacks plastics, fabrics and rubber. It is inactivated by organic matter, proteins and cationic detergents. Its range of action is wide and is popular for rapid disinfection in cases of spilled cultures and inactivation of unknown pathogenic strains.

Formaldehyde is most active in the gaseous form, specially in humidity conditions above 60% rh at 18 °C. 10% methyl alcohol helps inhibit polymerisation; 2% Borax inhibits corrosion. It is inhibited by ammonia, morphine, proteins and organic matter. The boiling method uses up 500 cc of formalin with 1 litre of water per 1000 cu.ft of space; the drip method uses 150 g of potassium permanganate with 280 cc of formalin. The disadvantage with both methods is that the vapours condense on cold surfaces. Formaldehyde fumigation is most effective at ambient temperature using an aerosoliser featuring special nozzles or the more popular revolving dispenser.

Metallic salts are effective antifungal agents for pretreatment of walls. They include copper sulphate, phenyl-mercuric acetate and phenyl-mercuric napthalate. Another commonly used fungicide is bromosalicylanilide.

Mites pose perennial problems in the tissue culture industry, and entry decontamination procedures include treatment with miticides. Common miticides are *Phosalone* (0.5%), *Mancozeb* (0.2%), *Endosulfan* (0.1%), *Monocrotophos* (0.05%) and *Neem seed kernel extract* (4%) in *Teepol* solution (0.1%).

Good Disinfection Practice: A Summary

The general principles are summarised here to serve as a guideline for the contamination control team. First decide on the type of disinfection programme. This requires consultation among the Microbiologist, Pharmacist and the User. Demand for disinfectants may come from many departments. There are also many sources of supply. All requests should be approved by the contamination control team, who can check whether they are appropriate and in conformity with the overall programme.

- List all purposes for which disinfectants are used, then check all requisitions and orders to ensure list is complete.
- Eliminate use of chemical disinfectants when an alternative can be reasonably employed. For example, when heat is an option choose sterilisation; or when thorough cleaning alone is adequate; or when disposable items can be economically used. This should then leave few remaining uses for disinfectant fluids.
- Select the smallest number of disinfectants possible for the remaining uses.
- Arrange for distribution of selected disinfectants at correct use dilution, or provide apparatus for accurate measurements at point of use.
- Make sure that every potential User of disinfectants receives adequate instructions on correct usage. These should include:
- The correct disinfectant concentration to be used for each task
- Substances that will react with, neutralise or otherwise interfere with the disinfectant
- The shelf life at the concentration supplied; the type of container and closure to be used; and the frequency with which the solution must be changed in use.
- Personal safety instructions: should gloves be worn? How to open and mix safely? What to do in case product comes in contact with skin or eye?
- The programme should be monitored to ensure that it is, and continues to be, effective. Periodic in-use tests, assays and estimations of concentration are recommended.

Disinfectants
Criteria for Selection

- Antimicrobial activity
- Solubility
- Stability
- Non-toxicity to human and animals
- Homogeneity
- Non-combination with extraneous organic material/ neutralisation
- Temperature
- Capacity to penetrate
- Desired concentration
- Time of exposure
- Bioburden level
- pH
- Moisture/ Humidity

Drawing up a Disinfection Programme

1. List all purposes for which disinfectants are used, then check all requisitions and orders to ensure list is complete.
2. Eliminate use of chemical disinfectants when an alternative can be reasonably employed. For example, when heat is an option choose sterilisation; or when thorough cleaning alone is adequate; or when disposable items can be economically used. This should then leave few remaining uses for disinfectant fluids.
3. Select the smallest number of disinfectants possible for the remaining uses.
4. Arrange for distribution of selected disinfectants at correct use dilution, or provide apparatus for accurate measurements at point of use.
5. Make sure that every potential User of disinfectants receives adequate instructions on correct usage. These should include:
   - The correct disinfectant concentration to be used for each task
   - Substances that will react with, neutralise or otherwise interfere with the disinfectant
   - The shelf life at the concentration supplied; the type of container and closure to be used; and the frequency with which the solution must be changed in use.
   - Personal safety instructions : should gloves be worn? How to open and mix safely? What to do in case product comes in contact with skin or eye?
6. The programme should be monitored to ensure that it is, and continues to be, effective. Periodic in-use tests, assays and estimations of concentration are recommended.

Properties and proper use of common disinfectants

Section	Property	Glutaraldehyde	Formaldehyde gas	Hypochlorite	H_2O_2	Alcohol ethyl	Iodophors	Chlorxylenol	QACs	Peracetic acid	Metallic salts	Phenolics
TYPE	Antiseptic	Y	N	N	N	Y	Y	Y	Y	N	Y	N
TYPE	Disinfectant	Y	Y	Y	Y	Y	Y	Y	Y	Y	N	Y
TYPE	Germicide	Y	Y	Y	Y	Y	Y	N	N	N	N	Y
USE	Additives	Y	Y	N	N	Y	N	Y	N	N	N	N
USE	Concentration (%w/v)	2	2-8	1	10	70	2	2	5	2	5	2
ACTIVITY	Fungi	E	G	P	F	E	G					
ACTIVITY	GPC	E	E	E	E	E	E	E	E	E	G	E
ACTIVITY	GNB	E	E	E	E	E	G	E	G	F	P	E
ACTIVITY	Spores	E	G	E	G	P	G	P	P	P	P	P
ACTIVITY	Lipid virus	E	E	E	E	E	G	G	G	G	F	E
ACTIVITY	Nonlipid virus	E	E	E	G	V	G	P	P	P	P	V
SUITABLE APPLICATIONS	Human tissue	N	N	N	N	Y	Y	Y	Y	N	N	N
SUITABLE APPLICATIONS	Hands & feet	Y	N	N	N	Y	Y	Y	Y	N	N	N
SUITABLE APPLICATIONS	Environment air	N	Y	N	N	N	N	N	N	N	N	N
SUITABLE APPLICATIONS	Contact parts	Y	N	Y	Y	Y	N	N	N	N	N	N
SUITABLE APPLICATIONS	Work surface	Y	N	Y	Y	Y	Y	Y	Y	Y	N	N
SUITABLE APPLICATIONS	Equipment surface	Y	N	Y	Y	Y	Y	Y	Y	Y	N	N
SUITABLE APPLICATIONS	Glassware	Y	Y	Y	Y	Y	Y	Y	Y	Y	N	N
SUITABLE APPLICATIONS	Culture spills	Y	Y	Y	Y	Y	N	N	N	N	N	N
SUITABLE APPLICATIONS	Walls & Ceiling	Y	Y	Y	Y	Y	Y	Y	Y	N	N	N
SUITABLE APPLICATIONS	Floor	Y	N	N	N	N	Y	Y	Y	N	N	Y
SUITABLE APPLICATIONS	Sinks	Y	N	Y	Y	N	Y	Y	Y	N	N	N
SUITABLE APPLICATIONS	Toilet	N	N	N	N	N	N	N	N	N	N	Y
INACTIVATED	Hard water	N	N	N	N	N	N	Y	N	N	N	N
INACTIVATED	Anionic soap	N	N	N	N	N	N	N	Y	N	N	N
INACTIVATED	Cationic detergent	N	N	Y	Y	N	N	N	N	N	N	Y
INACTIVATED	Cork	N	N	N	N	N	N	Y	Y	N	N	N
INACTIVATED	Organic matter	N	Y	Y	Y	Y	N	Y	Y	Y	Y	N
INACTIVATED	Proteins	Y	Y	Y	Y	Y	N	Y	Y	Y	Y	N
CHARACTERISTICS	Shelf life > 1 week	N	Y	N	N	Y	Y	Y	Y	Y	Y	Y
CHARACTERISTICS	Corrosive	Y	Y	Y	Y	Y	Y	N	N	N	N	N
CHARACTERISTICS	Attacks plastics	Y	N	N	Y	Y	Y	N	N	N	N	Y
CHARACTERISTICS	Stains	Y	N	N	Y	N	Y	N	N	N	Y	Y
CHARACTERISTICS	Residues	N	Y	N	N	N	N	N	N	N	Y	Y
CHARACTERISTICS	Irritate skin/eye/nose	Y	Y	Y	Y	N	N	N	N	Y	Y	Y
CHARACTERISTICS	Toxic	Y	Y	Y	Y	N	N	N	N	N	Y	Y
CHARACTERISTICS	Safe handling	N	N	Y	Y	Y	N	N	N	N	N	Y

Characteristics of Halogen Releasing Disinfectants

	Effective Concentrations, Contact Times	Advantages	Disadvantages	Examples of Uses
Chlorine Compounds: Sodium hypochlorite solution [1] (liquid bleach)	100-10,000 ppm (.01-1%) free chlorine 10-60 minutes (>= 3,000 ppm for broad spectrum)	broad spectrum inexpensive widely available bactericidal at low temperature	toxic, corrosive to skin and metals unstable at optimum effective pH of 6 inactivated by organic matter deteriorates under light and heat shelf life of dilutions is less than 1 week	general disinfectant waste liquids surface decontamination emergency spill clean up instrument disinfection
Calcium hypochlorite[2] granules, powder, tablets	as for liquid bleach	as for liquid bleach but more stable	as for liquid bleach above, except shelf life is longer	as for liquid bleach
NaDCC[3] (Sodium dichloroisocyanurate) powder, granules, tablets	as for liquid bleach	more stable than hypochlorites stable at pH 6.0	toxic, corrosive inactivated by organic matter	as for liquid bleach
Chloramine-T[4] (Sodium tosylchloramide) powder or tablets	as for liquid bleach	more stable, less affected by organic matter than hypochlorites longer activity than hypochlorites	deteriorates under humidity, light and heat	as for liquid bleach
Chlorine dioxide[5]	demand-release of chlorine dioxide in situ	longer activity than other chlorine compounds less corrosive, less toxic than other chlorine compounds effective at pH 6-10	aqueous solutions decompose under light	instrument disinfection gas sterilization of germ-free animal chambers
Iodine Preparations: Iodophors[6]	30-1,000 ppm (.003-.1%) free iodine 10-30 minutes	broad spectrum germicidal over a wide pH range generally nonstaining, less toxic and less irritating than aqueous or alcoholic iodine solutions	not consistently sporicidal efficacy reduced by organic matter some iodophor solutions support growth of *Pseudomonas*[7]	germicidal soaps and antiseptics surface decontamination work surface wipedown instrument disinfection

Notes

1. a 1/10 dilution of 5.25% bleach provides 5,250 ppm available chlorine
2. "high tested" provides 70-72% available chlorine; chlorinated lime or bleaching powder provides approximately 35% available chlorine
3. appproximately 60% available chlorine
4. approximately 25% available chlorine
5. To avoid shipping of this extremely reactive product, reagents ("base" and "activator") from commercially available kits are mixed with water to generate chlorine dioxide immediately prior to use
6. 10% povidone-iodine provides 1% available iodine
7. An iodophor stock solution may actually be a less effective germicide than its dilution. For example, a full-strength (10%) solution of povidone-iodine provides approximately 10 times less free available iodine than a 1/100 dilution. Iodophors must be used at the manufacturer's recommended concentrations.

Characteristics of Non- Halogen Releasing Disinfectants

	Effective Concentrations and Contact Times	Advantages	Disadvantages	Examples of Laboratory Uses
Alcohols	70-80% ethanol 60-95% isopropanol 10-30 minutes	low toxicity rapid action low residue non-corrosive	rapid evaporation limits contact time flammable, eye irratant may damage rubber, plastic, shellac ineffective against bacterial spores	skin disinfectant (antiseptic) surface decontamination benchtop, cabinet wipedown
Phenolic Compounds	400-50,000 ppm (.05-1.5%) 10-30 minutes	tolerant of organic load, "hard" dilution water leaves an active residue (may be desirable on some surfaces) biodegradable	pungent odour, corrosive, some forms toxic not sporicidal; limited activity against viruses leaves a residual film (undesirable in culture systems) may support growth of bacteria[1]	instruments and equipment disinfection disinfection of floors and other surfaces antiseptic soaps and lotions
Quaternary Ammonium Compounds	500-15,000 ppm (.05-1.5%) 10-30 minutes	combined detergent and germicidal activity stable working dilutions have low toxicity	non sporicidal, limited activity against viruses, mycobacteria most formulations not readily biodegradable may support growth of bacteria[2]	surface decontamination equipment wipedown antiseptic formulations available floors and walls
Hydrogen Peroxide	3-30% aqueous solution 10-60 minutes 6% for 30 minutes may kill spores	rapid action no residue low toxicity environmentally safe	limited sporicidal activity corrosive to some metals potentially explosive at high concentrations stock solutions irritating to skin and eyes	surface decontamination instruments and equipment
Peracetic Acid (PAA)	.001-.3% aqueous solution gas phase: 2-4% 5-120 minutes	broad spectrum sporicidal at low temperatures can tolerate organic load rapid action nontoxic decomposition products leaves no residue	pungent odour corrosive to some metals shelf life of dilutions is less than 1 week stock solutions irritating to skin and eyes stock must be protected from heat, light gas phase: respiratory irritant, fire hazard above 55°C	instruments and equipment gas phase sterilization of chambers for germ-free animals

Characteristics of Non- Halogen Releasing Disinfectants

	Effective Concentrations and Contact Times	Advantages	Disadvantages	Examples of Laboratory Uses
Aldehydes:				
Glutaraldehyde	0.5-2.5% alkalinized aqueous solution 2-30 mins; up to 12 hours to kill all spores	broad spectrum does not corrode metal can tolerate organic load	expensive pH, temperature dependent pungent odour toxic: skin, eye, respiratory tract irritant activated solutions have less than 2-week shelf life	cold sterilant and fixative surface decontamination instruments, equipment, glassware
Formalin (37% aqueous formaldehyde)	3-27% formalin (1-10% formaldehyde) in 70-90% alcohol 10-30 minutes	broad spectrum inexpensive does not corrode metal can tolerate organic load	pungent odour skin, eye and respiratory tract irritant potential carcinogen (animal studies) may require 24 hrs or more to kill all spores	cold sterilant and fixative surface decontamination instruments and equipment
Formaldehyde (gas)	1-3 hours	as for formalin effective penetration	as for formulin flammable porr penetration of covered surfaces	on site decontamination of biological safety cabinet HEPA filters enclosed areas
Ethylene Oxide Gas	50-1200 mg/L 1-12 hours	broad spectrum no heat or moisture evolved penetrates packaging materials	flammable, reactive toxic: potential carcinogen and mutagen some sterilized items may need more than 24 hours for outgassing	heat or moisture sensitive supplies, instruments and equipment

Fumigation & Surface Disinfection Methods

Formaldehyde		
Conditions:	Humidity	60% to 80%
	Temperature	Low, approx. 18°C
Additives:	Inhibit polymerisation	10% methyl alcohol
	Inhibit corrosion	2 % Borax
Neutralisation		Ammonia in shallow tray
Fumigation of Rooms		
Gaseous/Fumes per 1000 cft		150g $KMnO_4$ + 280 ml formalin
Boiling/fogging per 1000 cft		500 ml formalin + 1000 ml water
Fumigation of Cabinets		
Boiling formalin per cft		2 ml
Vaporise paraformaldehyde per cft		0.3 g
Surface disinfection		1:10 formalin
Hydrogen peroxide		
Additives		Silver nitrate
		Antimony nitrate
		60% IPA
General use		2 - 10% in distilled water / 60% IPA
Fumigation:	By fogging	20 % H_2O_2 in distilled water
Surface disinfection		5 - 10% H_2O_2 in distilled water
Water decontaminatlon		100 ppm H_2O_2 + 2 ml Formalin
Virus inactivation		50% H_2O_2
Virosil		
Fumigation:	By fogging per 1000 cft	200 ml in 800 ml of distilled water
Surface disinfection		5% in distilled water

Media for isolation

Plate count agar for bacterial solution

Potato dextrose agar/ Sabroud's agar for fungal isoaltion

Afterword

There may have been very little in this presentation about which you had little or no prior knowledge, or could not have deduced by yourself with a little effort. It is not so much a question of how much we know, as how much of our knowledge and capabilities we bring to practical use on a day to day basis.

For example, when we read something, whether technical or otherwise, we often encounter words we do not comprehend. (Just as a matter of curiosity, can you remember when you last opened your dictionary?). Yet how many of the words we know and understand do we use in our day to day communications?

"Concept" and "awareness" percentages are often high; but when it comes to "practice" percentages are low. The success of this presentation lies in how well it has motivated you to start *applying* your knowledge to usher in improvements in your own micro-contamination control programme.

To help you get started, I have included a small check list of things you could attempt to improve your work site.

Good Luck with your microcontamination control initiatives!

Things you could do to improve your work site

Microcontamination control audit report

1. Item (s)/person(s) found coming into/leaving cleanroom
   (a) without authorisation,
   (b) with authorisation but avoidable

2. Item (s)/person(s) in cleanroom
   (a) without authorisation
   (b) with authorisation but avoidable

3. Any loop detectable in material/personnel/process flowpath

4. Avoidable movements of men/material identifiable?

5. Undue frequency of entry and exit of any person observed?.

6. Any suggestions for improving
   (a) isolation of critical space
   (b) doorways and door movements
   (c) entry barriers and staging operations
   (d) airflow distribution
   (f) task related cleanliness
   (g) qualification programme, including airflow visualisation, sedimentation counts, surface sampling

7. Any recommendations for improving:
   (a) gowns, gowning and laundry
   (b) code of conduct within cleanroom
   (c) bioprofiling each operator
   (d) sanitation programme
   (e) disinfection agents and methods

True or false: The Answers

1. ***Cleanrooms are contaminant free environments***

   By their very classification, cleanrooms admit presence of contaminants. For example, the cleanest is ISO Class 1, where we still allow one suspended contaminant of size 0.1 micron or larger per cubic metre of air sampled, and several more of smaller sizes. A cleanroom is at best a zone where there are control measures to cope with such contaminants with reasonable confidence of preventing them from contaminating the product.

2. ***A cleanroom is incomplete without an air shower***

   Unless you can "validate" the air showering process and establish beyond all doubt that the air showering reduces the person-borne contaminant density by a consistent, repeatable and reproducible factor, the air shower will continue to be an unqualified add-on, desirable but not proved to be essential. The onus of proving that it does the job it is purported to do lies with you.

3. ***HEPA filter is a 0.3 micron bacteria tight sieve. Larger particles are arrested; smaller particles escape.***

   The MPPS (maximum penetrating particle size) is 0.3 micron for a HEPA; but it is not a sieve Its efficiency is higher on either side of its MPPS. The fact that the viable count downstream of the HEPA is not always zero confirms that the odd bacteria can escape once in a way, although the large majority do get trapped.

4. ***Particle count at 0.5 micron or larger per cubic foot of air sampled immediately downstream of a properly installed new HEPA filter should always be 100 or better***

   If the upstream contaminant density is above prescribed limits, the count can be higher, though nothing is wrong with the filter or its installation.

5. ***LAF refers to air moving at 90 fpm in parallel lines.***

   Though the Orange Guide continues to refer to "laminar" flow, the ISO Standards use the term "unidirectional" airflow. The airflow fields should be non-intersecting, not necessarily in straight parallel lines. The Orange Guide indicates the velocity range as 90 +/- 20 fpm, the ISO allows a greater latitude from 40 - 100 fpm. In practice, air velocities sometime go as high as 140 fpm and are still deemed to be within the "laminar" range.

6. ***A HEPA can have an "acceptable" leak.***

   The "acceptable" penetration is also referred to as the acceptable "leak"

7. ***A HEPA may be repaired at site if the media is damaged.***

   Yes, subject, of course, to the limits specified in the IEST Recommended Practice Guidelines.

8. ***It is not important whether the measurement is taken with an airborne particle counter sampling at 0.01, 0.1 or 1 CFM, because readings are automatically extrapolated.***

   Readings from instruments sampling below 1 CFM is at best a rough estimation, because they may not have the suction power to draw in larger suspended particles

9. ***If airflow is reduced, pinhole leaks are detected more easily.***

   If there are pinhole leaks in the media, penetration will increase with decreasing airflow, relatively independent of particle size. This is because the constriction of airflow through a pinhole is a function of the air velocity whenever the constriction of airflow through the fibrous filter media. Therefore, at 20% or one-fifth of full test flow, a pinhole shows up as 5 times greater in proportion to total flow than it does at full flow. Also, at higher velocities particles impact upon the fibres of the filter element directly, whereas at lower velocities Brownian motion causes them to drift and wander. In the process they are more likely to find their way out of the leak.

   Another reason is that ss airflow reduces, the leakage of the challenge aerosol through the pinhole causes an increases in the concentration downstream. The "masking" effect caused by surrounding "clean" airstreams is less pronounced,.

10. ***At the end of a properly validated sterilisation cycle all microorganism are dead.***

    All inactivation processes cause an exponential decay from the initial bioburden, and the process asymptotically approaches zero, but never ever becomes zero. This is why we have concepts like PSI (Possibility of Survivor Index) and SAL (Sterility Assurance Level). An SAL of 10^{-6} means you have reduced the bioburden to one viable survivor in a million.

Center for GMP *(formerly P3QUEST)*
49 Aruna Enclave Trimulgherry, Secunderabad 500015
Voice: 27791629 **Fax:** 27992912
eMail: cgmp@vsnl.com **URL:** business.vsnl.com/cgmp

Mr C K Moorthy is the Founder and Principal Facilitator of Center for GMP, which seeks to address the long felt need in our country for a credible, knowledgeable and reliable agency that offers cost-effective, meaningful, and ready-to-use solutions, insights, guidance and counsel to empower Users of controlled environments, so that their facilities, practices and procedures remain in step with current national and international norms.

Center for GMP conducts full-scale public Workshops of 2-day and 3-day durations from time to time at Hyderabad; and also offers at-site structured training, which are designed as modules and aimed at different levels of target audience.

Our workshop seeks to supplement, not *supplant*, Users' own in-house training initiatives. This Structured programme combines a judicious blend of lectures, OHP transparencies and short relevant videos. The emphasis is on interactive group dynamics and discussions centering around real life problems. By explaining the *Whys*, *Hows* and *Whats*, it avoids the *Do it this way because I say so* approach.

The workshop is designed to be in step with cGMP expectations for personnel training and features pre- and post- training tests, performance appraisal and related documentation, including Certificate of Participation.

Why attend the cGMP Workshops?

- Growth in production volumes magnifies associated risk of rejects
- Ensuring consistency and homogeneity in product quality across multiple manufacturing facilities, both in-house and contracted
- Need for developing and retaining quality personnel
- Professional orientation for new inductees and *floaters*
- Safety net for protection when trained employees quit
- Continuing education for those well experienced and trained
- Nudge *experts* and *veterans* who have been too tied up with routineto implement changes for improvement

More information about us, our vision and mission, forthcoming programmes and activities, and feedback from clients may be gleaned from our website.

Glossary

As in every other field, microcontamination control too has, over the years, developed its own lexicon, words that have meanings peculiar to the field. A partial list of such words is given here; others may be found in the section *Terms and Definitions* featured in every guide and standard.

50% count — If a particle counter is calibrated for measuring a particular size, say 1μ, it will detect all particles of that size and larger. If challenged with an aerosol containing a normal (Gaussian) distribution of particles whose count median value is 1μ, it will detect only 50% of that population, since the remaining 50% would be below the calibrated size threshold.

Aerosol generator — A device for generating an aerosol

Aerosol photometer — A light scattering mass concentration indicator. (Instruments of this type have a threshold sensitivity of at least 10^{-3} μg per litre for 0.3μ diameter DOP particles and are capable of measuring concentrations over a range of 10^5 times the threshold sensitivity.)

Air shower	An enclosed cubicle in which high velocity streams of filtered air from nozzles on walls and ceiling help remove loose lint or grit from gowned cleanroom operators prior to their entry into the critical zone. More often than not, it has only cosmetic value, and gives rise to an undue sense of security and complacency.
Air curtain/Barrier	Air moving downwards at high velocity to segregate two adjacent areas by acting as a barrier for cross movement of air between them. At 600 fpm (as measured at 1 metre height from floor) this serves effectively as a thermal barrier, isolating an air-conditioned zone from one that is not; at 1600 fpm it helps prevent ingress of flying insects. It is ineffective against crawling insects. The turbulence at floor level, kicking up settled dust, renders it unsuitable for installation near cleanrooms.
Airborne particulate	The level of cleanliness specified by the maximum allowable *cleanliness class* number of particles per cubic metre of air (or cubic foot of air), as determined by the statistical methods laid down in relevant sections of the Standard 209E. The name of the class in SI units is taken from the logarithm (base 10) of the maximum allowable number of particles, 0.5μ and larger, per m^3. The name of the class in English (US customary) units, as used in prior editions of Fed Std 209, is taken from the maximum allowable number of particles, 0.5μ and larger, per cu.ft.
ALARA	As low as reasonably achievable, an acronym in mass photometry, that advocates minimal concentration of challenge aerosols, so that test filters are not unduly loaded.
APC	Aerodynamic particle counter, also known as time of flight counters, that determine particle size by the time it takes to traverse between two points in the sample cell under controlled drag conditions.
Anisokinetic sampling	The condition of sampling in which the mean velocity of the flowing air stream differs from the mean velocity of the air entering the inlet of the

	sampling probe. Because of particle inertia, anisokinetic sampling can cause the concentration of particles in the sample to differ from the concentration of particles in the air being sampled.
As-built cleanroom	A cleanroom (facility) that is complete and ready for *(facility)* operation, with all services connected and functional, but without equipment or operating personnel in the facility.
As specified	When the terms *as specified* or *shall be specified* are used without further reference, the degree of control needed to meet product requirements will be specified by the User or contracting agency.
At-rest cleanroom	A cleanroom (facility) that is complete, with all services *(facility)* functioning and with equipment installed and operable or operating, as specified, but without operating personnel in the facility.
Calibration	Comparison of a measurement standard or instrument of unknown accuracy with another standard or instrument of known accuracy to detect, correlate, report or eliminate by adjustment any variation in the accuracy of the unknown standard or instrument.
Clean air device	A clean bench, clean work station, wall or ceiling-hung module, or other device (except a cleanroom) which incorporates HEPA/ULPA filter(s) and motor-blower(s) for the purpose of supplying clean airflow to a controlled work space.
Clean workstation	A clean workstation is a work bench or similar working enclosure characterised by having its own filtered air or gas supply.
Clean zone	A defined space in which the concentration of airborne particles is controlled to meet a specified airborne particulate cleanliness class.
Cleanroom	A room in which the concentration of airborne particles is controlled and which contains one or more clean zones. (Compare how this definition differs from the earlier one given in previous

versions of the standard: *A cleanroom is an enclosed area employing control over the particulate matter in air with temperature, humidity, and pressure control, as required. To meet the requirements of a "cleanroom" as defined by this standard, all cleanrooms must not exceed a particulate count as specified in the air cleanliness class as defined.)*

CMD — Count median diameter, or diameter of that particle which represents the median of that population which is being counted. If the population of particles in a given aerosol has more fines that gross particles, the CMD will be closer to the smaller size end of the spectrum.

CNC — Condensation nucleus counter, an instrument for counting small airborne particles, approximately 0.1μ and larger, by optically detecting droplets formed by condensation of a vapour upon the particles.

Chance positive result — Sensing a leak where none really exists, causing false alarm.

Chance negative result — Missing a leak where one exists, giving a false sense of security

Coincidence error — When a larger particle obscures one much smaller in size while counting, causing the counter to miss out on the latter

DOP, air generated — A heterogeneous (polydispersed) aerosol generated by blowing air through liquid dioctylpthalate, (generally referring to di-2-ethyl-hexyl-pthalate, technical grade) at room temperature. When generated with a Laskin type nozzle, the approximate light scattering mean droplet size distribution is: 99+% $< 3\mu$, 50+% $< 0.7\mu$ and 10+% $< 0.4\mu$

DOP — An aerosol generated by quenching (condensing) vapour that *(thermally generated)* has been evaporated from liquid DOP by heat. The aerosol has a light scattering mean diameter of 0.3μ with a geometric standard deviation of about 1.4.

Dynamic range	The ratio between the largest and smallest detectable values in an instrument
ED	Equivalent diameter. Suspended particles are not always regular spheres. For purposes of sizing, scientists have evolved formulae for assigning equivalent sizes for different irregular shapes. The equivalent diameter is the diameter of a reference sphere having known properties and producing the same response in the sensing instrument as the particle being measured.
Entrance plane	A plane perpendicular to the unidirectional airflow located immediately upstream of the region of interest (typically the work area unless otherwise specified) and having the same dimensions as the cross section of the clean zone perpendicular to the direction of the airflow.
Fallout count	Number of particles that settle down or fall from the air in the environment. These are the particles that could contaminate.
First air	The air which issues directly from the HEPA filter.
First work location	The work location nearest the downstream side of the HEPA filters in a laminar airflow device.
Forward scattering	Any particle, no matter how big or small, scatters light that impinges on it. This scattering is in all directions. The pattern of the scatter in the forward (with source of light behind) and near-forward directions is an important indicator that correlates with the size of the particle causing it.
GMD	Geometric mean diameter. If the aerosol has a population of *n* particles, the GMD is the *nth* root of the product of the diameter of the individual particles. If there are more fines, the GMD will be closer to the smaller size end; if there are more of larger particles, the GMD value will be closer to the bigger size end.

Grade 1 Filter (HEPA/ULPA): Fire resistant construction throughout, complying with the minimum requirements of UL 586.

Grade 2 Filter (HEPA/ULPA): Semi-combustible filter with noncombustible media, but either separators (in case of some HEPAs), frame, or both made from combustible material, complying with minimum requirements of UL 900 Class 2.

Gravimetric concentration: A term in photometry that refers to the aerosol concentration as measured by weight.

HEPA Filter: A throwaway extended media dry type filter in a rigid frame with a minimum efficiency of 99.97% for 0.3μ thermally generated DOP (or specified alternative) aerosol particles, and a maximum clean filter pressure drop of 2.54 cms d'eau (1" wc) when tested at an airflow of 100% of the rated flow capacity.

Isoaxial: A condition of sampling in which the direction of the airflow into the sampling probe inlet is the same as that of the unidirectional airflow being sampled.

Isokinetic sampling: The condition of isoaxial sampling in which the mean velocity of the air entering the probe inlet is the same as the mean velocity of the unidirectional airflow being sampled.

Isopleths: Points in space with identical suspended contaminant density.

Laminar airflow: For the purpose of our discussion, laminar airflow is defined as airflow in which the entire body of air within a confined area essentially moves with uniform air velocity along parallel flow lines.

Laminar airflow cleanroom: A room in which the laminar airflow characteristics predominate throughout the entire airspace, with a minimum of eddies.

Laminar airflow	A work station in which the laminar airflow characteristics *clean work station* predominate throughout the entire airspace, with a minimum of eddies.
Laskin nozzle	A special design of nozzle used for the generation of a heterogeneous DOP aerosol by compressed gas.
LOD	Limit of detection, or smallest value sensed and read by an instrument.
Micron (micrometer, μ)	A unit of measurement equal to one-millionth of a meter, or approximately 0.00003937 inch.
MMD	Mass median diameter. Though small particles may be many, the mass of the larger particles is disproportionately significant, and the MMD represents the diameter of that particle that stands as the median in the population when arranged in a cumulative mass order. This explains why there is often such a wide difference in the values of the CMD and MMD.
Monitoring	The routine determination of airborne particle concentrations as well as other relevant conditions, in cleanrooms and clean zones.
Nonunidirectional	Airflow which does not meet the definition of unidirectional *airflow* airflow; referred to as "turbulent" or "nonlaminar" airflow in prior editions of the Federal Standard.
Nonlaminar flow	A room supplied with filtered air with no specified *cleanroom* requirement for uniform airflow patterns or uniform air velocity.
Nonlaminar flow	A work station characterised by nonuniform air patterns and *clean work station* velocities. This includes work stations which have constricted air exhaust or ports.
Operational cleanroom	A cleanroom (facility) in normal operation, with all services *(facility)* functioning and with equipment and personnel, if applicable, present and performing their normal work functions in the facility.

OPC	Optical particle counter
Owl	An optical instrument for visual measurement of the particle diameter of a monodispersed aerosol.
Particle	A solid and/or liquid object generally between 0.001μ and 1000μ in size.
Particle concentration	The number of individual particles per unit volume of air.
Particle size	The apparent maximum linear dimension of a particle in the plane of observation observed with a microscope, or the *equivalent diameter* of a particle detected by automatic instrumentation. *[Compare this with the definition in prior editions: Particle size is expressed as the apparent maximum linear dimension or diameter of the particle.* *Note: While measurements from light scattering equipment may vary some from maximum linear dimension, this variation is not usually considered significant for normal cleanroom monitoring requirements.)]*
Parallel airflow	Unidirectional airflow, as demonstrated by introduction of an isokinetic smoke stream which exhibits a measured dispersion of not more than 14^0 from straight line flow.
PEL	Permissible exposure level, a term relating to acceptable safety levels of toxic vapours and fumes.
Penetrometer	A self-contained instrument for the determination of penetration characteristics of very high efficiency filter media and filter units with thermally generated DOP in accordance with Mil-Std-282.
Photometric	A term in photometry that refers to the aerosol concentration *concentration* as measured optically
Prefilters	A filter to trap gross particulates located upstream from and with lower collection efficiency than the HEPA filter. The efficiency of initial prefilters is usually in the 20-30% range by the NBS Discolouration (Dust Spot) Test while intermediate prefilters usually have a collection efficiency of 80-90% by the same test.

Probing or scanning	A method for disclosing and determining the exact location of leaks in filter units in which the probe nozzle of an aerosol photometer is held approximately 2.54 cms (1”) from the area to be tested, and moved at a rate of not more than 3.05 m/min (10 fpm) across the test area. For best results, the airflow rate is 20% of the rated capacity of the filter under test.
SPC	Single particle counter, an instrument such as an optical particle counter or a condensation nucleus counter, capable of resolving responses from individual particles.
Suspended count	Count of particles that remain suspended in air.
TLV	Threshold limiting value, a term relating to acceptable safety levels of toxic vapours and fumes.
Total recovery method	When a HEPA or ULPA is inaccessible for probing at its leaving face, the concentration measured downstream can confirm a leak (due to detection of excess penetration); but the exact location of the leak cannot be identified.
Tyndall effect	Scattering of light by an aerosol.
Type A (HEPA)	A HEPA filter that has been tested at rated flow with thermally generated DOP smoke, and whose efficiency in the encapsulated form is 99.97% on 0.3μ particles.
Type B (HEPA)	A HEPA filter that has been tested for overall penetration at 100% rated flow, and at 20% rated flow with thermally generated DOP smoke, and whose efficiency in the encapsulated form is 99.97% on 0.3μ particles.
Type C (HEPA)	A HEPA filter that has been tested for overall penetration at 100% rated flow with thermally generated DOP smoke, and whose efficiency in the encapsulated form is established as 99.97% on 0.3μ particles. In addition, it is probed for leaks by scanning at 20% rated flow using cold polydispersed DOP aerosol generated at room temperature using a Laskin type nozzle and no detectable leaks are found to be present.

Type D (ULPA) — An ULPA filter tested as per procedure for Type C HEPA, except that the filter efficiency is a minimum of 99.999% on 0.12μ particles.

Type E (ULPA) — An ULPA filter that has been designed, constructed and tested in strict accordance with Mil-F-51477 (Military specification for fire *resistant* filters for biologic use) or Mil- F-51068 (fire *retardant*).

U-descriptor — The maximum allowable concentration (particles per cubic metre of air) of ultrafine particles. The U-descriptor serves as an upper confidence limit and/or the upper limit for the location averages, as appropriate.

ULPA — Ultra low penetration air filter, a throwaway extended media dry type filter in a rigid frame having minimum particle collection efficiency of 99.999% for particulate diameters 0.12μ and larger in size.

Ultrafine particles — Particles in the size range of approximately 0.02μ and larger. Ultrafine particles are operationally defined by the relationship for counting efficiency *vs* particle size.

Unidirectional airflow — Airflow having generally parallel streamlines, operating in a single direction, and with uniform velocity over its cross- section; referred to as "laminar" airflow in prior editions of the Federal Standard.

Uniform airflow — Unidirectional airflow pattern in which the point-to-point readings are within $\mp 20\%$ of the average airflow velocity for the total area of the laminar flow work zone.

Upper confidence limit — An expression from statistics, which refers to the upper limit *(UCL)* of the estimated mean which has been calculated so that, in a specified percentage of cases, its value exceeds the true population mean, both means having been sampled from a normal (Gaussian) distribution. In the US Fed Std 209E, a 95% UCL is used.

Verification The procedure for determining the compliance of air in a cleanroom or clean zone to an airborne cleanliness class limit and/or U-descriptor, as specified.

Volumetric A term in photometry that refers to the aerosol concentration *concentration* as measured by volume.

Work zone The volume within the cleanroom which is designated for clean work and for which testing is required. The volume shall be identified by an entrance and exit plane normal to the airflow (where there is laminar airflow).

9 789386 819604

Printed at Repro India Ltd.